From The Ground Up

How Frontline Staff Can Save America's Healthcare

Peter Lazes
Marie Rudden

16pt

Read How You Want
LARGE PRINT BOOKS, BRAILLE & DAISY

Copyright Page from the Original Book

From the Ground Up

Berrett-Koehler Publishers, Inc.
1333 Broadway, Suite 1000
Oakland, CA 94612-1921
Tel: (510) 817-2277, Fax: (510) 817-2278
www.bkconnection.com

Ordering information for print editions
Quantity sales. Special discounts are available on quantity purchases by corporations, associations, and others. For details, contact the "Special Sales Department" at the Berrett-Koehler address above.
Individual sales. Berrett-Koehler publications are available through most bookstores. They can also be ordered directly from Berrett-Koehler: Tel: (800) 929-2929; Fax: (802) 864-7626; www.bkconnection.com
Orders for college textbook/course adoption use. Please contact Berrett-Koehler: Tel: (800) 929-2929; Fax: (802) 864-7626.
Distributed to the U.S. trade and internationally by Penguin Random House Publisher Services.

2020-1

Book producer: Westchester Publishing Services; Text designer: Westchester Publishing Services; Cover image: Rick Finkelstein; Cover designer: Peggy Archambault; Peter Lazes photo: Marie Rudden; Marie Rudden photo: Peter Lazes.

TABLE OF CONTENTS

Dedicated to our children and grandchildren

Foreword

Think back to the last time you were really sick. Perhaps you had a high fever and cough, or severe abdominal pain and vomiting, or you were in a car accident. Remember that feeling of vulnerability, of fear, of not being sure what to do or what would happen to you.

At the moments when we are sick, we desperately need a health system that is both competent and caring, that is armed with today's medical knowledge but that also treats us with kindness and respect. It needs to speak our language, understand our spiritual natures, and respect our family structures.

I remember when I was hit by a car and had a broken leg and spent a day at a fine health center, where I was well treated by the doctors and the nurses, until I hobbled on crutches to where I was to have my pre-op labs. As I walked in the door and smiled at the receptionist, she said in a harsh voice, "You know we are closed 12 to 1p.m. for lunch." It was such a trivial thing, but upset by the car accident, fearful of the upcoming surgery, tired from using the crutches, I sat down feeling so sad and defeated in the waiting room.

Of course, everyone needs a lunch break. Were I running that system, I may have suggested staggering lunch breaks, but that really wasn't the issue: I was just overwhelmed. Had she just said, "I'm so sorry, you will have to sit and wait an hour because the nurses are at lunch," I would have been fine. But when we are sick or injured, we lack the reserve that buffers us from unkind words at other moments.

That's why this book is so important. For our healthcare system to meet our needs, we must engage, promote, support, and inspire the frontline workers—the nurses, the doctors, the pharmacists, the phlebotomists, the physician assistants, the receptionists, the aides, the security guards, and the environmental staff—to care for our patients. They are the ones providing the care. They are the ones who know what changes are necessary in order to improve care. Everyone else should be eliciting their ideas and supporting their efforts.

Two major supporters—the unions who represent workers and the administrators of the hospitals—are often mistakenly at odds with one another despite sharing a common goal: high-quality healthcare. This goal can be achieved only though respecting and listening to employees.

I have had the good fortune in the cities where I have worked—San Francisco, Los Angeles, and now New York City—to partner with enlightened labor leaders and hospital administrative colleagues to improve the healthcare for public hospital patients. Although the localities vary, the important ingredients of this work, well-illustrated in this book, consist of engaging frontline workers and collaborating, with an open heart and shared-power paradigm, with labor leaders and others who genuinely care how to make healthcare both competent and kind.

I hope that as you read this book, you will not only learn the successful techniques of engaging and supporting frontline staff but also be inspired to improve healthcare wherever you work.

Mitchell H. Katz, MD
CEO and president, NYC Health + Hospitals

INTRODUCTION

Uprising

> Using your workforce as an engine for innovation is critical for our economy. Who knows better about what makes a quality operation than folks who are in the front lines?
>
> —*Thomas Perez, former U.S. Secretary of Labor*

Although the massive civil outburst following the 1968 assassination of Martin Luther King Jr. had taken place more than five years before I, Peter Lazes, started to work in Newark, New Jersey, I could still smell the smoke of the burned-out buildings on Central Avenue from my office at New Jersey Medical School.

It was as if that uprising had just ended when I started my new job, developing a community psychiatry program for the patients at Martland Hospital, the large city hospital served by the medical school's interns and medical residents. Most of the stores on Central Avenue had remained untouched since they were set on fire during the massive civil response to Dr. King's murder. Promises made by Mayor Kenneth Gibson, the first black mayor of any major northern city, to rebuild Newark and to provide better healthcare services for its citizens, remained unfulfilled. Community activist Amiri Baraka responded to this failure with censure and disappointment, stating that Gibson's attention was primarily focused on "the profit of Prudential, Port Authority, and huge corporations ... while the [community] residents were ignored."[1]

Eventually, New Jersey Medical School's departments of Community Medicine, Internal Medicine, and Psychiatry began to hire practitioners like me to work with the mayor and with community groups to improve healthcare services for Newark residents. I found that by focusing on what patients were experiencing as they waited for and received clinic or emergency care, and by listening to observations of the staff who helped them—from laboratory staff to receptionists, nurses, LPNs, aides, and Emergency Department (ED) physicians—I could assist in devising a care system that worked better for all involved. Ever since then, I have spent my career devising methods to help frontline staff, workers, and administrators collaborate on improving the systems to which they devote their lives.

As this book approaches publication, the COVID-19 pandemic has been escalating daily around the world. The method that we espouse here is thus particularly relevant. Hospital staff have an imperative need to be involved in ordering equipment, setting up isolation areas, and determining staff ratios in order to keep themselves and their patients safe.

The Growing Chasm between Administration and Frontline Staff

From 1980 to 2016, I was a member of the faculty at Cornell University in the School of Industrial and Labor Relations. This position provided me the opportunity to consult with a variety of organizations, helping them to keep jobs in the United States while improving working conditions for their employees and the quality of their products and services. For the past 20 years, I have focused particularly on healthcare systems as a researcher, educator, and consultant to medical centers and nursing homes from New York City to Los Angeles. These experiences have made me aware of practical and effective methods that can improve healthcare services in our country.

My work in Newark from 1972 to 1978 brought me into early, intimate familiarity with the challenges facing urban healthcare and mental health treatment systems. Sadly, 40 years later, I continue to witness our healthcare delivery systems—the organizations of people, institutions, and resources delivering healthcare services to meet the needs of target populations—being plagued by the same struggles, and still routinely producing poor patient outcomes at high cost. To a large extent, this arises from patients' limited access to adequate preventive and diagnostic care and from a lack of integrated patient services, especially for those with chronic, stigmatized, or complex conditions.[2] These problems persist in large cities, but the systemic difficulties also affect rural and suburban communities, with rural areas especially afflicted by the scarcity of operating hospitals and physicians. I have noticed that fragmentation of care tends to go hand in hand with an alienated staff and with an administration that focuses less on patients and their needs and more on the workings and demands of an institutional hierarchy. Indeed, the growing need for hospital administrators to focus almost totally on insurance reimbursements and on meeting state or federal regulations has led to a growing chasm between them and the clinicians who directly provide patient care within many organizations.

This chasm has led to an increasing experience of frustration and even despair among those nurses, physician assistants, and doctors who care for patients. Ross Fisher, whose internal medicine practice centered on the outpatient care of patients with complex chronic diseases, describes this tragic situation: "From everything I read and hear about, I should be one of the most sought physicians to meet today's patient population needs. But our current broken healthcare system fails to respect and accommodate the requirements necessary to succeed in managing these challenging patients, and the reality today is that I am marginalized and diminished in capacity by forces removed from my influence." He describes those forces especially as including the fact that in most settings, "the power to dictate how much time a provider spends with a patient is divorced from the primary ... caregivers."[3] In addressing this dilemma, Massachusetts governor Charlie Baker stated, "Our system should reward clinicians who invest in time and connection with patients and families."[4]

No matter what form of payment is used so that all Americans have access to healthcare services—whether one has insurance through his or her employer, exercises a public option, or is enrolled in Medicare for All—we need to *restructure our delivery systems* and *pay for clinicians to have sufficient time with their patients.* As it currently stands, in most U.S. hospital and outpatient settings, caregivers have become increasingly despairing about the degree to which their time with their patients is managed by administrators and insurers. As they mourn their ability to be clinically effective, this dramatically affects their patients' healthcare experience.

How the System Disconnects Clinicians from Patients

I, Marie Rudden, MD, have worked as a practitioner in multiple medical settings for the past 50 years, and for the past 10 I myself have suffered from two complex chronic illnesses (systemic lupus erythematosis and Sjogren's syndrome), an experience that has illuminated the shortcomings of the American healthcare system quite vividly and personally for me. As clinicians in even excellent tertiary care institutions have little time allotted for patients with complex conditions, I have had to become my own advocate, pointing out aspects of my history about which my doctors have little time to inquire, and communicating test and consultation results myself to each of the specialists involved in my care. As a practicing physician, I am prepared for this task. However, I have seen firsthand among my own patients with chronic illnesses how bewildering this process is for those without a medical degree. I routinely call their multiple specialists in order to understand my patients' diagnoses and treatment strategies, and then translate what I find to answer their questions.

I have been able to do this because I am in the minority of remaining physicians who have practiced privately and thus control their own schedules—a sadly vanishing breed, due to the increasing, expensive incursions into practice by insurers and regulators starting in the late 1980s, which have driven physicians into working within group practices and larger hospital systems. These incursions began with the limitation by Medicare on physicians' charging for more than one intervention per day, which keeps doctors from visiting their patients whom they have just admitted to the hospital, to follow up on their care. It prevented me from seeing patients with psychiatric emergencies, first by themselves and then later in the day with their families, whose support they required in order to avoid hospitalization.

This situation accelerated with the spread of HMOs, which restricted many other aspects of patient care. I well remember an untrained "behavioral healthcare representative" instructing me to refer a quite troubled patient to an online support group rather than approving her continued treatment with me. It took hours of my time to appeal this foolhardy decision.

Further, since the enforcement of a universal requirement that clinicians record every visit through an electronic medical records system, primary care doctors now spend nearly two hours typing into these records for every hour they spend in direct patient care![5] The time these records systems require drives clinicians *away* from fully listening to their patients and from communicating with other specialists.[6] As one nurse reported, "I didn't become a nurse in order to collect data."[7] While electronic records were partially intended to help coordinate patient care through the sharing of information from clinical visits, lab tests, and procedure results, their use has become the bane of most clinicians' work lives. Most EMR programs require them to follow a rubric that often fails to include central issues addressed within their patient visits. Our healthcare system must be reorganized so that clinicians have enough time and resources to practice more humanely and effectively without such intrusions.

The Purpose of This Book

As both of us have been occupied in our careers with what makes organizational systems more effective and have observed the central role of frontline staff and caregivers in this effort, we offer methods for restructuring healthcare systems in a way that makes collaboration and active communication among administrators, medical staff, and patients a key value. This book explores exactly what it takes to effectively engage staff and providers in improving the patient care shortcomings within their institutions. We do this by presenting case studies of institutions that have successfully implemented major systemic changes in this manner, by reviewing research findings and outcomes, and by conveying the direct words and experiences of staff who have participated in changing their healthcare organizations.

We offer several avenues toward redressing care system shortcomings but focus particularly on the use of Labor-Management Partnerships to restructure care as it is currently offered. Such partnerships are based on a cooperative engagement among administrators, providers, and staff; offer contractual protections for each group; and include defined methods for initiating and overseeing unit-based, departmental, and system-wide changes. The outcome of an effective, well-resourced Labor-Management Partnership can be more meaningful work for employees, greater workplace morale, increased awareness for administrators of flaws in their operating system, improved patient care, and cost savings.

Throughout this book, we examine questions such as: How can the knowledge and communication gaps between administrators and those who offer care be overcome in our healthcare systems? What roles do management and healthcare union leaders (when applicable) need to play to capture the knowledge and firsthand experience of their frontline staff in making decisions about the practice of patient care? What interventions are most useful for assisting them in turning their ideas into workable proposals? What processes and structures best accomplish effective changes within a given healthcare system? And what are the challenges that arise in involving frontline staff and their unions, when pre sent, in redesigning their healthcare delivery system?

We have shaped this book around the specific methods that healthcare systems can employ in order to enlist their frontline staff in diagnosing and rectifying difficulties in providing high-quality patient care. This book not only is a manual detailing what can be achieved when frontline staff have a direct voice in controlling their practice environments, but also was written to provide a method for accomplishing transformative changes in how our hospitals and outpatient clinics work.

All Americans deserve and should have access to high-quality, affordable healthcare services delivered by professionals who know them and who have sufficient time and resources to care for them.

Why Healthcare Systems?

Much has been written about the need for healthcare reforms in America. Governmental attention is usually directed to increasing citizens' access to insurance, to rewarding institutions for positive outcomes, or to penalizing institutions for practices that fall short—for example, for frequent and early hospital readmissions. This top-down approach has been valuable in focusing hospital and systems administrators on essential bottom-line markers of effective treatments. Such approaches, however, need supplementation by finer-gauged methods for identifying and addressing the service gaps particular to each institution.[8]

The participation of frontline staff in identifying areas of concern, and in creating and, most important, implementing changes that will transform our current systems, is vastly underutilized, even as it has been shown to assist hospitals and health systems in becoming more efficient and delivering higher-quality outcomes. One study by Anita Tucker at Boston University, using data from 20 hospitals, documented that frontline staff proposals for improving patient safety were more effective than those originally offered by the institutions' managers and also led to more effective utilization of staff time and efforts.[9]

North American hospital administrators are rarely taught in business, medical, nursing, or public health schools how to meaningfully engage with clinicians or caregiving staff or with the unions that represent healthcare workers.[10] To the detriment of all, clinicians and other frontline staff are essentially told, "Keep your thoughts about patient care and the work environment to yourself. We know what's best to keep this institution afloat." This situation is particularly unfortunate in healthcare organizations, in which nurses, aides, pharmacists, dietary and cleaning personnel, physician assistants, and physicians can all observe problems in care delivery, in cost excesses, and in the uses of technology, and can contribute to solving them. When implemented effectively, frontline staff participation creates a cogenerated process,[11] weaving together the knowledge and skills of frontline staff *and* management to result in a stronger organization. We offer practical examples of how to implement and sustain an effective participatory process, as well as an analysis of the challenges in undertaking such a change process.

Focusing this book on healthcare organizations is also particularly important, as this is a growing sector of our national economy, and one that elicits significant concern due to skyrocketing costs and limited access to high-quality services. Healthcare costs now consume over 18 percent of our current gross domestic product (GDP),[12] and the healthcare sector is expected to generate more new jobs than most segments of the economy, at least through 2026.[13] The need for more coordinated, cost-effective services is also growing due to an aging population with patients who may have complex, intersecting illnesses such as diabetes, hypertension, autoimmune disorders, pulmonary diseases, and cardiac diseases.

Since healthcare services are mostly provided directly to patients on-site, aside from radiology and pathology, they cannot be outsourced,[14] which is a cost-cutting strategy used in other sectors of the U.S. economy. Thus, healthcare organizations must find different ways to cut costs while also providing high-quality-of-care outcomes. It makes intrinsic sense for frontline providers and staff, who daily witness the aspects of their system that may not be cost-effective, to be enlisted in a joint effort toward cost containment.

The Importance of Labor-Management Partnerships

In the United States, unions represent 20.7 percent of the healthcare sector's workforce, a statistic that is increasing[15] just when union membership is shrinking in most other segments of our economy.[16] Our focus on employee participation within healthcare needs to take this fact into account. Happily, many unions representing healthcare workers[17] have themselves become increasingly sophisticated in working with healthcare administrators to create joint labor-management participation processes.

Modern healthcare organizations—outpatient clinics, inpatient settings, nursing homes—interface constantly with an array of insurance companies, each with its own set of cost-monitoring practices, as well as with state and federal regulatory agencies. As stated earlier, the need for these organizations to stay on top of the ever-changing regulatory and reimbursement processes has led to an increasing stratification within them, with CEOs, CFOs, and whole administrative branches devoted to budgeting and regulatory issues rather than to what happens within the hospital: patient care.[18] In fact, from 1975 to 2010, "[t]he number of healthcare administrators increased 3,200 percent. There are now roughly 10 administrators for every doctor within United States healthcare systems."[19] In such top-heavy organizations, administrators have become too far removed from the daily process of patient care to effectively manage all the issues that arise within their complex medical settings.[20]

Complex organizations, as a rule, face real difficulty in making changes effectively and efficiently due to their having to face multiple variables, often occurring within siloed departments. It has become a common understanding in in the organizational studies literature that in complex institutions, the flexible but structured involvement of all key stakeholders is required to achieve an optimal result.[21] For healthcare organizations, this means that the staff who interact with and directly care for patients must be involved in decision-making processes—in analyzing both care-delivery shortcomings and opportunities for improvement. Working together, administrators and frontline staff can claim responsibility for envisioning, researching, and implementing the changes necessary to create a high-functioning complex organization devoted to caring for sick patients (see figure 1). At the unit and departmental levels especially, this involves consultation and knowledge sharing with all contributors to their particular mission.

Figure 1. Healthcare Facilities Are Very Complex Organizations

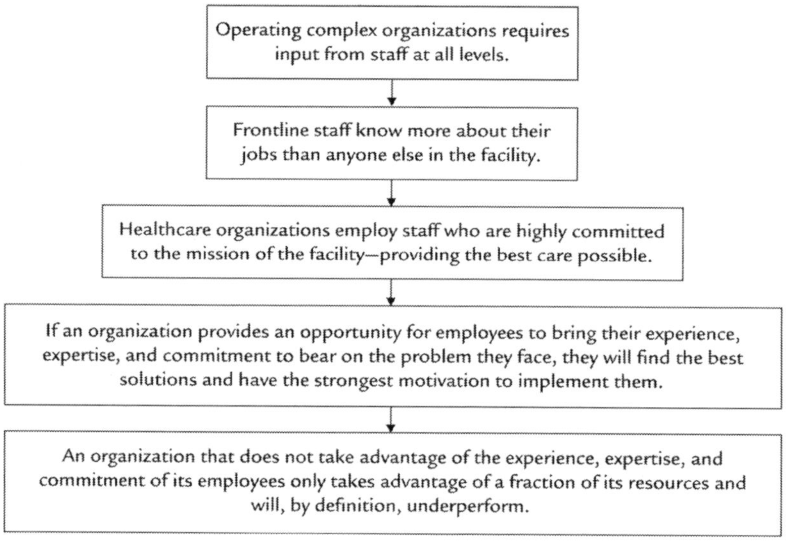

The Labor-Management Partnership approach has emerged as especially useful in formalizing processes through which frontline staff can contribute to improving their workplaces while also making their own working lives more meaningful. The approach creates a clear process for frontline staff and administrators to jointly identify and solve patient care problems, make work decisions, and implement their solutions. We focus in this book on defining and demonstrating the use of this strategy.

Examples of the use of Labor-Management Partnerships to structure a shared decision-making process among the organizational stakeholders are provided throughout the book. Within such partnerships all stakeholders, including patients, contribute to and benefit from this process (see figure 2).

One example of a Labor-Management Partnership, described in detail in chapter 4, concerns the joint effort of administrators, nurses, physicians, and other staff in one hospital to respond to a series of sudden deaths that occurred within their cardiology unit over a short time period. The hospital administration's initial response to this crisis was to penalize nurses who had not responded quickly enough to the patients' cardiac monitors. A more forward-thinking response occurred when the hospital's Labor-Management Partnership created a joint task force composed of clinical personnel on the unit and their departmental administrator to study what had actually led to these errors. As a result of their joint analysis of the crisis, the hospital eventually purchased a more effective cardiac monitoring system, and various practices surrounding the transport of monitored patients and the assignment of nurses to high-risk patients were instituted. As a result, no more such deaths occurred in subsequent years. The administration alone had not been aware enough of the practical difficulties in caring for and monitoring such patients to be able to arrive at such a solution by themselves.

How This Book Is Organized

Although our book focuses on the importance and application of healthcare Labor-Management Partnerships to improve patient outcomes and control healthcare costs, the basic principles presented can and should apply to other economic sectors as well. *From the Ground Up* begins with a brief review of employee participation activities and Labor-Management Partnership practices as they evolved in the United States (chapter 1) and in Europe (chapter 2). These histories are presented from the vantage point of a practical analysis: What were the goals of such activities? How were their processes structured? What sorts of problems did these activities attempt to address? What outcomes were obtained? These chapters orient the reader to the particular practices of Labor-Management Partnerships, which can deepen and extend earlier employee involvement activities.

Figure 2. Healthcare Partnerships Can Benefit *All* Stakeholders

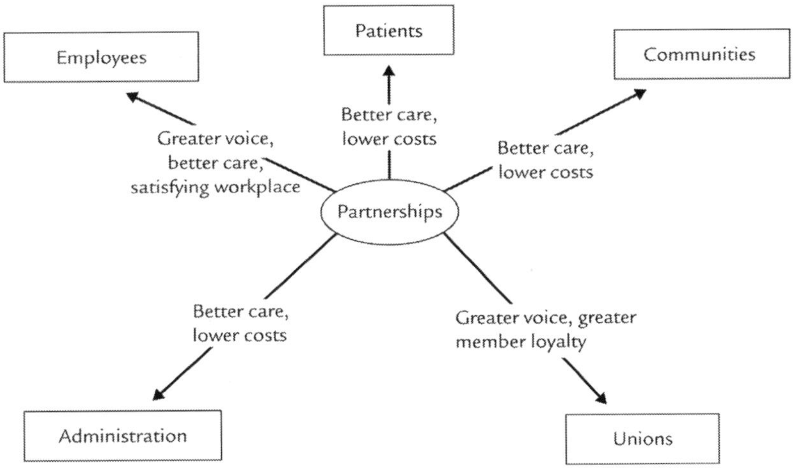

Chapter 2 also highlights the critically important connection between worker participation and increased civic participation among frontline workers, an issue amplified in chapter 8. This is crucial for our country today, given the alienation too many citizens feel toward their local and national government.

Chapter 3 presents specific core practices for developing and sustaining a viable Labor-Management Partnership. Two extensive case studies are employed to illustrate these necessary practices, which include creating a social contract between labor and management about their mutual goals, with protections for each side and a clear decision-making process; developing educational activities for both staff and senior leaders about the need for, and processes involved in, change; improving overall labor relations within the organization; using sector strategies to find solutions already in use in other venues; and documenting results of the change processes.

Chapter 4 describes structures for effectively implementing frontline staff participation within Labor-Management Partnerships. Unit-based and departmental approaches can achieve both process and quality-improvement outcomes within current work systems, while the Study Action Team approach can create new work structures that address cost-saving and quality improvement throughout the organization. Vignettes from both healthcare and manufacturing partnerships pre sent the pros and cons of each of these approaches, providing a broad understanding of which form of partnership might best suit a particular workplace.

Chapter 5 details ways in which work group leaders can respond to departures from a work focus in their teams and suggests approaches to problems that can arise in teams when members occupy different places in the organizational hierarchy or come from different cultural backgrounds.

Chapter 6 details how labor unions can foster a worker participation process, offers advice to union leaders who are contemplating engaging in such activities, and describes the risks and benefits to labor unions for engaging in such activities.

Chapter 7 offers suggestions for healthcare leaders seeking to expand existing Labor-Management Partnerships. The first section of this chapter focuses on two unique approaches to enlist greater frontline staff participation within the existing work systems;

the second section describes a method borrowed from the technology industry for launching new Partnerships that significantly transform current delivery systems. We also discuss the need for Partnerships to include patient as well as staff input in their proposals for systemic change and suggest a method for the Partnerships to interface with insurance companies regarding reimbursement changes.

Chapter 8 summarizes the successes of Labor-Management Partnerships but also takes a close look at what has happened when existing Partnerships that offered initial promise were not sustained. We describe preventive measures based on these findings. We also document research on the increase in civic participation among workers and staff who participate in Labor-Management Partnerships, a finding that is of crucial importance to sustaining our democracy.

In the epilogue, we reprise the importance of worker participation as a critical process for improving healthcare outcomes. We also emphasize the central concepts and strategies offered in the preceding chapters, most of which are highly practical. We summarize the state of our current healthcare "system" in which chaotically intertwined for-profit systems entangle clinicians' abilities to deliver adequate care to their patients. Finally, we issue a *call for collective action* to all healthcare administrators, professionals, and frontline staff to challenge these systems. We outline ways in which the corporations that currently hold patient care systems hostage can be pressured, through political and staff group actions, to resurrect the value of "first, do no harm" in treating patients.

In sum, this book will inform you about the historical development of approaches for engaging frontline staff in job redesign and in the creation of more effective organizational systems. The book gets you under the covers, so to speak, exploring what it *really* takes to effectively initiate, implement, and sustain employee involvement activities. It demonstrates how Labor-Management Partnerships particularly can help organizations to evaluate the effectiveness of their current systems and to design more functional structures. We emphasize too the importance of establishing collaborative leadership processes to engage and sustain employee participation efforts.

PART ONE

Background

CHAPTER 1

The Evolution and Value of Labor-Management Partnerships

> In the long history of humankind (and animal kind too) those who learned to collaborate and improvise most effectively have prevailed.
>
> —*Charles Darwin*

"Environmental services workers want to know the effect our work has on patients and their visitors. We also want to offer suggestions about changing what isn't working," William Quintana, an environmental services employee at Maimonides Medical Center, in Brooklyn, New York, thus described his motivation to work in a Labor-Management Partnership (LMP) there. A tall, burly, somewhat quiet man, Quintana had made suggestions throughout his first year at Maimonides about ways to improve hospital cleanliness. His supervisor ignored these ideas, but his union steward took notice of them and recommended that he be included in a Study Action Team about hospital cleanliness being formed by the Maimonides LMP. By that point, Quintana was reluctant to join, as he had already felt unheard and was not convinced that he would be listened to now. However, he was persuaded to participate in the team's process and became increasingly enthusiastic about it. Along with other housekeeping staff, Quintana collected and examined outcome data about their work on maintaining a clean hospital, proposed a detailed plan to increase their effectiveness, and took responsibility for implementing their suggested changes. "Now we are getting access to follow-up information to make sure that our plan is working,"[22] he emphasized proudly in an interview conducted after his group finished their work. The results of their study included a 25 percent reduction in housekeeping employee absenteeism, a 75 percent increase in patient satisfaction with hospital cleanliness, and an approximately 45 percent savings on housekeeping supplies. Empowered by the respect he experienced during the Study Action Team process, Quintana decided to return to college, became involved in coaching other LMP teams, and eventually was elected as a union shop steward at Maimonides.

Quintana's work and that of his team exemplifies the benefits of Labor-Management Partnerships for quality improvement, cost savings, and job satisfaction in hospital environments (see table 1). The Labor-Management Partnership in which they worked represents the product of an evolution in collaborative methods between workers and managers that has developed in the United States since the 1950s.

Evolution of Labor-Management Collaborative Efforts in the United States

Developing formal ways to unleash the intelligence, knowledge, skills, and imagination of frontline staff has improved the productivity and effectiveness of U.S. organizations since the start of World War II.[23] The history of employee participation in the United States is important, as these activities have established a strong and effective foundation for current approaches to improving healthcare delivery systems and other organizations.

The history of employee participation and eventual development of Labor-Management Partnerships in the United States began with Walter Reuther, a tool and die maker and former head of the General Motors (GM) division of the United Auto Workers (UAW) union. Reuther espoused a broad vision for the role of labor in the American economy. He felt that although the primary job of the union was to protect workers and to improve their economic situations, it also had a primary obligation to strengthen the U.S. economy and simultaneously bring greater dignity to workers.[24]

Table1. Significant Outcomes of Labor-Management Partnerships

Organization	Outcomes
C. F. Hathaway Shirts	Saved 400 jobs by implementing a new manufacturing process. Eliminated rework and reduced costs by upward of 35%.
Los Angeles County Depart-ment of Health Services	Increased patient satisfaction scores to over 91%.
	Diabetic education increased by 96%.
	Created Patient-Centered Medical Homes to coordinate the care for all patients using county health facilities.
	Creating a just culture workplace—encouraging staff to identify patient and staff safety issues.
Kaiser Perma-nente	Organized unit-based teams in all facilities, enabling frontline staff to identify and solve crucial problems.
	Created an electronic medical records system.
Maimonides Medi-cal Center	Reduced patient falls by 50%.
	Turnaround time for lab results reduced to 30 minutes from two to three hours.
	Cost reductions for housekeeping supplies of 40%.
	Reduced response time to cardiac monitors to under one minute.
	Achieved medication reconciliation in all major depart-ments.
Saturn Corpora-tion	Designed and manufactured a competitive small car costing less than Japanese model.
Tarrytown GM plant	Moved from last place to first in production quality within its division.
	Reduced grievances from 2,000 to 32.
University of Ver-mont Medical Center	Setting new staffing levels in all departments.

Organization	Outcomes
Xerox	Saved 180 jobs by creating new production methods saving $3.2 million in operating costs.

To this end, he and other union leaders became strong advocates of employee participation processes to accelerate production of aircraft and tanks during World War II. Workers in the automotive industry believed that the quickest way to produce planes for the war effort was to manufacture them in automobile plants. "Time will not permit us to wait until new mass production factories for aircraft and aircraft engines finally swing into action. Emergencies require short-cut solutions. This plan is labor's answer to a crisis,"[25] Reuther said in 1940. Reuther's "500 Planes a Day" proposal created a blueprint for converting auto plants into factories manufacturing planes. His plan included sustaining wages at current levels and agreeing not to strike, in order to maintain labor peace during the war. President Franklin D. Roosevelt had made known his interest in having labor advise him about domestic manufacturing as the war was being waged, so Reuther's plan was well received by the key administrators responsible for building military aircraft.[26]

Although the automotive unions' war efforts were successful, enthusiasm in the United States for labor participation in managerial decisions faded with the dawning of the McCarthy era, the "Red Scare," and the Cold War with the Soviet Union. The idea of promoting workers' participation or increasing the role of unions in the workplace now met with suspicion and hostility as being communist-inspired. Discouraged, unions retreated to their traditional roles of collective bargaining, defending workers' jobs, and representing workers in grievance hearings: roles that became increasingly predictable, entrenched, and static.

By the 1970s, however, American political culture had changed enough that the idea of workers' participation in redesigning their jobs regained acceptability. A new breed of management scholars had begun to advocate for job enrichment and work-enhancement activities. They saw these approaches as important for reducing workers' alienation by allowing workers to control their work pace (job enhancement) and to expand some of their job responsibilities (job enrichment).[27] At this time, UAW leaders such as Irving Bluestone, vice president of the union's GM division, also began to advocate for creation of more meaningful work for their members, in addition to better pay and more generous benefits.

Bluestone understood that the workforce wanted more from their jobs than just a paycheck. Many workers felt aggrieved by monotonous working conditions and by their inability to alter work practices they knew were wasteful or could be accomplished more efficiently. Bluestone's articulation of the need for more gratifying work for his members coincided with the new academic concepts of job enrichment and enhancement.

Gary Bryner, president of the UAW 1112 at the GM assembly plant in Lordstown, Ohio, described the problem of worker alienation before the U.S. Senate's Subcommittee on Employment, Manpower, and Poverty on July 25, 1972:

> There are symptoms of the alienated worker in our plant—the absentee rate has gone continually higher. Turnover rate is enormous. The use of alcohol and drugs is becoming a bigger and bigger problem. So has apathy within our union movement towards union leaders and towards the Government.... [The worker] has become alienated to the point where he casts off the leadership of his union, his Government. He is disassociated with the whole establishment. That is going to lead to chaos.[28]

Rising up against alienating working conditions, the union went on strike at the Lordstown assembly plant in 1972. Its members wanted a voice in decision making in their workplace. After the monthlong strike, workers won greater opportunities to choose their jobs, to change jobs on a regular basis, and to select the equipment and supplies they used on the assembly line. The Lordstown strike received national attention due to the unusual nature of the workers' demands. More recently, the 2019 Chicago teachers strike focused on class size and services for students, not just on wage increases.[29]

After the Lordstown strike, the quality of work life, and not simply adequate wages and benefits, became for the UAW a critical requirement of future contracts with management. Bluestone hoped that similar outcomes could be achieved elsewhere:

> U.S. management has always paid lip service to the idea that it is the people performing the work who are the most important in the production process. As a matter of fact, however, the treatment given the workers has belittled the worker.... Management should cooperate with the workers to find ways to enhance the human dignity of labor and to tap the creative resources of each human being in developing a more satisfying work life, with emphasis on worker participation in the decision-making process.[30]

In 1974, Bluestone identified a potential site for a quality of work life initiative. At a GM plant in Tarrytown, New York, a receptive plant manager, labor relations executive, and local union president were willing to consider starting such a project, which would give workers a role in decision making about the effectiveness of their jobs as they were currently structured. Although labor relations at this plant were poor, and management "acted like despots to employees,"[31] Bluestone considered the Tarrytown plant a good site because of the visionary leadership of its local union president and because a new plant manager wanted to work with the union in a new way.[32] All the key players agreed that they needed to try to work together differently, hoping perhaps to set an example for the industry.

Bluestone became the project broker. His life's purpose, again, focused on enriching the lives of workers, their families, and their communities. "Only a strong labor movement can preserve democracy," he contended. "The first thing Hitler did was to destroy the labor parties in Germany."[33] Doug Frazer, then the president of the UAW, crystalized Bluestone's role in advocating for increased worker participation: "Unlike the rest of us, who tended to be screamers, he had tremendous patience with management. I used to get impatient with his patience."[34] Bluestone convinced the Tarrytown local union president that a quality of work life initiative could improve his members' working conditions. "We as a union knew that our primary job was to protect the worker and improve his economic life. But times had changed, and we began to realize we had a broader obligation to the workers—to become more involved in decisions affecting their own jobs, to get their ideas, and to help to improve the whole quality of life at work beyond the paycheck,"[35] reasoned the Tarrytown local UAW president.

Quality of work life activities, exemplified by the Tarrytown effort (described shortly), constituted an early approach to collaboration between labor and management in the United States. These activities aimed primarily at increasing productivity and creating more meaningful jobs, although many activities improved the processes and quality of production within the industry.

What follow are details of the evolution of worker participation activities in the United States.

Approach #1: Quality of Work Life Initiatives

The first step of the 1972 Tarrytown plant Quality of Work Life (QWL) initiative was the formation of two problem-solving teams to find solutions to difficulties in the quality of their production process. Both workers and managers had observed significant inefficiencies and quality issues in the trimming and glass-sealing operations at the plant. Flaws in these operations were resulting in water leaks through car windows and trim during rainstorms and problems of glass breakage.

After initial problem-analysis training, each team of five frontline workers, meeting weekly, quickly located the origins of the production problems that caused the leaks. Plant engineers had not been able to solve this problem previously. Because these initial teams succeeded in resolving the water leakage, an agreement was reached to train all plant employees in basic problem-solving skills and to establish more teams to address other production issues. To assist workers in these new problem-solving teams, management made critical production information available, data never previously shared with hourly employees.[36] All teams received time off from their production jobs to work on resolving the various quality issues. Their meetings lasted an hour every week or every other week, based on the importance of the issue they were addressing.

Within four years after establishing the QWL initiative, the Tarrytown plant went from one of the poorest in quality (measured by inspection counts and dealer complaints) to one of the best in an 18-plant division. Besides repairing water leaks, another important quality problem that a QWL team addressed successfully was reducing window glass breakage.

Implementing the QWL process at the Tarrytown plant decreased absenteeism from 7.3 percent in 1970 to 2.5 percent in 1978, while the number of grievance complaints between workers and managers fell drastically during those years from 2,000 to only 32.[37] Unfortunately, in 1974, management initiated two series of layoffs because of the OPEC oil crisis, which decreased General Motors car sales. Nonetheless, QWL teams continued to improve the quality of the cars they produced, and absenteeism remained at a reduced level. Tarrytown's impressive results encouraged the UAW to establish similar QWL activities at Ford and other GM assembly plants.

QWL programs such as the one at Tarrytown gained increasing popularity in the late 1970s and '80s. Hundreds of these initiatives were implemented at

AT&T with the Communications Workers of America, in the steel industry with the United Steelworkers, in men's and women's apparel plants with the Amalgamated Clothing and Textile Workers Union and the International Ladies' Garment Workers' Union, and in some schools and state government offices with the American Federation of Teachers and the American Federation of State, County and Municipal Employees.

Greenberg and Glaser summarized QWL activities as "process[es] by which an organization attempts to unlock the creative potential of its people by involving them in decisions affecting their work lives."[38] Dick Walton, another researcher tracking the development of QWL activities, offered a similar definition: "An organization responds to employees' needs by developing mechanisms to allow them to share fully in making the decisions that define their lives at work."[39] Walton stressed that QWL opens communication channels between labor and management to help build mutual trust.[40]

QWL activities gave workers the ability to tackle problems in their immediate work areas as well as in their departments. The problem-solving teams established through QWL initiatives resembled the *quality control circles* (QC circles) that had already become highly successful in Japan for improving product quality, particularly in the auto industry. QC circles comprised groups of 5 to 15 frontline staff who received training in problem solving and quality improvement skills, as well as in documenting their results. The Japanese used QC circles to balance the command-and-control management structures in their plants with a self-governing process that they believed would enhance quality outcomes.[41] QC circles helped Japanese manufacturing companies outperform their American counter parts during the late 1980s and '90s.

Although similar to QC circles, the QWL activities adopted in the United States tended to include unions as partners in overseeing development of the problem-solving teams, including selection of team members, choice of relevant work areas, and ensuring effective team training.[42] QWL activities also tended to seek not only to solve production or work unit problems, but also to improve workers' job satisfaction and job commitment. Employee participation activities such as QWL initiatives and Labor-Management Partnerships often do achieve that, as the dramatic reduction in Tarrytown absenteeism and the cases of William Quintana and others suggest.

Approach #2: Quality Improvement Activities

By the early 1980s, increasing competition from countries such as Japan, plus customer demands for better-quality products and services, began to place considerable pressure on North American manufacturers. To respond to these demands, companies needed to find ways to reduce costs and bring products to market faster. One strategy toward these ends was the creation of more structured worker participation processes to improve services and products system-wide and cut costs while still creating meaningful work for employees.[43]

An example of this shift in focus of worker participation activities occurred in the early 1980s, involving the Amalgamated Clothing and Textile Workers Union at the Xerox Corporation. Xerox, like many other manufacturing companies, started their worker participation process by establishing problem-solving teams at the four plants in Webster, New York, which then manufactured all Xerox machines. These teams were initially patterned largely on QC circle practices, rather than employing the QWL processes described previously.[44]

Although highly effective in Japan, QC circles (QCC) were difficult to implement in the United States. A study by S.G. Hayward concluded that this was because senior management was often not committed to full employee participation, because a process that was fully under management control alienated employees, and because QCC goals seemed only vaguely connected to overall company strategies.[45] In traditional QC circles, unlike in QWL teams, unions and frontline staff had no role in overseeing the change process and had limited ability to choose which problems to address.

In 1980, the first year of Xerox employee involvement activities, this was essentially the case. Within a year, however, senior management and union leaders became aware of the limitations in their problem-solving team approach and resolved to improve it. These leaders, along with technical staff and assembly line workers, engaged in sessions to analyze the problems with their participation process. Peter Lazes, co-author of this book, consulted at these meetings, which concluded that to more fully engage frontline workers in their teams, they needed to be involved in choosing the problem areas to study, as they were detecting significant production issues that were being neglected.

It was recognized, in fact, that a much larger set of production issues needed to be studied in order to help Xerox maintain its market share: shortening the time it took to bring products to the market, improving the quality of products and customer service, and reducing the cost to customers of copiers, paper, and toners. The group chose to adopt Lazes' suggestion, as their consultant, to begin a targeted Labor-Management Partnership process for this expanded endeavor.

All the stakeholders would participate in hammering out its specific goals and ground rules. Within the Partnership, the union would have the ability to co-determine[46] critical areas for investigation and problem solving as well as responsibility for selecting problem-solving team members. Union leaders created the innovative practice of using frontline workers with particularly good communication skills and problem-solving team experience as internal coaches and trainers for the new teams.

In addition to these ground rules involving the union, an employment security clause (in the form of a sidebar agreement[47]) guaranteed that no employee would lose her or his job as a result of changes brought about by Labor-Management Partnership activities.[48] This agreement was critical in arresting workers' fears that these activities might result in layoffs as a primary cost-saving solution. Other activities were established to support the Labor-Management Partnership, to ensure that it would become "the way we work" at Xerox. These included distributing a bimonthly newsletter updating all employees on outcomes of the different problem-solving teams, conducting a yearly conference to share and spread best practices throughout the company, and creating an annual review process for managers and supervisors to evaluate the extent to which they promoted employee participation activities in their departments. Another innovation was that problem-solving teams became responsible for implementing their own solutions to production issues.

Over a three-year period, all Xerox employees in the four manufacturing plants who volunteered to become members of problem-solving teams were trained in problem-solving tools, in running effective meetings, in cost-benefit analysis, and in conflict resolution.

Meanwhile, each plant formed a Labor-Management Planning and Policy Committee and a Xerox Division Labor-Management Planning Committee to help identify plant-or system-wide problems on which to focus.[49] These Xerox Labor-Management Planning and Policy Committees had the authority to create interdepartmental workgroups to tackle problems requiring several departments to work together. Meanwhile, many other labor-management teams at Xerox continued to focus on improving the quality of Xerox machines in their particular department.[50]

The creation of Labor-Management Partnerships in the early 1980s, then, represented a shift from approaches in which teams of employees solved very real but isolated production problems to the broader process of improving manufacturing quality and reliability within an entire system.

The Xerox Labor-Management Partnership process resulted in improved quality of new and refurbished Xerox machines and in methods that brought the new models to market faster. The U.S. Department of Labor circulated news of the impact of Xerox's Labor-Management Partnership work nationally and internationally, and it became a model for future Labor-Management Partnership work, ultimately replicated in many other organizations.[51] Its success eventually resulted in an overall shift from undertaking quality of work life activities without an overlying, systemic focus and structure, to embedding such activities within a Labor-Management Partnership with clear goals, ground rules, staff, and a bud get.

Influenced by existing manufacturing company QWL activities, some hospital systems had begun to focus on unit-based problem-solving activities to improve patient care and create more meaningful work. In 1997, Kaiser Permanente developed its Labor-Management Partnership (LMP) process, one of the first in healthcare organizations along with the LMP at Maimonides Medical Center mentioned earlier. The LMP at Kaiser established a basic contract for joint work between its unions and managers, budgeted for Partnership activities, and hired staff as internal consultants and researchers.

In recent years, the Partnership has focused on providing frontline staff with opportunities for making changes in their departments about patient care and safety, as well as the implementation of a new medical records system and of community support programs for patients. Unit-based teams at Kaiser have also worked on such projects as developing a safe lifting process for nursing staff and reducing needle sticks, a significant staff safety issue. Kaiser teams have focused, too, on creating better shift-to-shift communications and on reducing hospital-acquired infections.

Other hospital systems that have adopted the unit-based team approach include the Maimonides Medical Center in Brooklyn, New York, and the

Allegheny Health Network in Pittsburgh, Pennsylvania. At Allegheny, unit-based teams have focused on such issues as improving handoffs between shifts, prevention of catheter-associated urinary tract infections, and prevention of central line–associated bloodstream infections. Practices that contribute to the success of such unit-based activities within Labor-Management Partnerships are described in more detail in chapter 3.

Approach #3: Transformative Activities to Create New Delivery Systems

While frontline staff teams have been quite successful at tackling discrete problems within and between hospital units and departments, they cannot address systemic issues in a hospital or healthcare delivery system. Different strategies are essential to create transformative changes in an entire organization's operation. In addition to employing unit-based and departmental strategies, Maimonides Medical Center and the Los Angeles County Department of Health Services each needed to enact systemic changes in order to create new, more effective delivery systems. They used two transformative approaches toward this end: *sector strategies* (at LA-DHS) and Study Action Teams (at Maimonides Medical Center). These approaches have been applied to underperforming organizations since the 1980s to enhance service quality while controlling costs and offering employees more meaningful work,[52] but they have only recently been employed within healthcare systems.

Sector strategies are research-proven best practices within a given industry that enable an organization to increase the performance of current systems. Using a sector strategy maximizes resources by using proven methods already in practice, rather than having each individual organization attempt to reinvent the wheel. Union and management leaders establish familiarity with the new strategies in their sector by conferring with colleagues in their industry (e.g., healthcare, automobiles, men's apparel, education) or, more commonly, by doing their own research to identify novel strategies within the sector. Consultants working with multiple organizations in a sector who become familiar with best practices can also be hired to educate the different stakeholders about them.

Although radically changing a production process or healthcare delivery system seems risky, having access to the outcomes of a proven sector strategy provides labor and management leaders with data to justify investing in a new approach.

The use of sector strategies has recently been an important element in improving patient care at the LA-DHS, as it was in improving quality and reducing costs at the C.F. Hathaway Company, a shirt manufacturer in Waterville, Maine, where co-author Lazes consulted in 1994. The latter consultation resulted in the first use of sector strategies in a Labor-Management Partnership process. Spurred by a management threat to close their plant, Hathaway union and management representatives, with myself as their consultant, met with the Harvard Center for Textile and Apparel Research to seek an alternative to relocation abroad. The Harvard group advised the delegation to adopt a new *modular manufacturing approach* as the best strategy for improving quality and reducing shirt manufacturing costs.

This method alters the traditional assembly line process, where each person performs one specific sewing job, to a system in which a group of workers assemble garments together in a more efficient manner. After extensive pressure from the union and from community organizations, Hathaway management agreed to implement this strategy instead of closing and relocating. The company's decision to adopt the modular manufacturing approach resulted in significant improvements in their shirt quality, in radical cost reduction, and in a more rapid plant adjustment to color, fabric, and design changes in their products.[53] This new manufacturing process enabled the Hathaway plant to remain open for eight more years after this intervention, until 2002 when it was closed, with all work outsourced.

At the Los Angeles County Department of Health Services, Dr. Mitchell Katz and other senior managers researched methods for improving patient access to treatment and for receiving coordinated care. They were particularly interested in data about Patient-Centered Medical Homes (PCMH), an important sector strategy for healthcare delivery systems, which were yielding extremely positive outcomes in improving patient access and the quality of patient care.[54] This system creates a permanent team of practitioners and specialists who see patients on a regular basis, rather than the traditional, impersonal L.A. County outpatient clinic approach, in which rotating practitioners never really got to know their patients. Besides providing them a consistent team of healthcare professionals, PCMHs enable patients with chronic illnesses to receive comprehensive care, with primary care providers following clear protocols.[55]

When fully implemented, this approach increases coordination between primary care and behavioral health services. Patient-Centered Medical Homes control healthcare costs by reducing emergency room use for routine care, by eliminating duplicative lab and radiological testing, and by helping chronic care patients avoid hospitalization through treating their conditions with regular visits to a primary care provider and specialists. Although departmental and unit-based problem-solving teams (continuous improvement teams) also have been used to improve basic services in LA-DHS ambulatory care facilities, adapting the PCMH approach was critical in creating more fully integrated services across departments. The Medical Home approach entailed practices ensuring that patients received needed supportive services within their community as a result of creating the position of care coordinators.

When a sector strategy isn't available and a work system needs significant changes,[56] the Study Action Team (SAT) process has been an extremely important tool in Labor-Management Partnerships. An SAT differs from unit-or department-based teams in offering a more intensive approach and a wider focus. A small group (usually six to eight) of employees, managers, and technical staff are freed full-time from their normal jobs for several months to investigate current operations and propose methods to address overall systemic problems. This analysis of the effectiveness of operations throughout an organization can radically redesign organizational work systems, resulting in significant changes in jobs, new operating procedures, and reassessment of which technologies to use. Implementing an SAT process can yield vast quality improvements and cost reductions. The Study Action Team process thus transcends the scope of work of traditional Labor-Management Partnerships that principally focus on improving existing systems.[57]

Similar to a sector strategy, the SAT process enables an organization to discover new ways of working without being constrained by current jobs, technology, work rules, and compensation systems.

In 1981, the Xerox Corporation used the SAT approach for the first time in North America at their Components Manufacturing Operations (CMO) in Webster, New York.

The union representing Xerox workers persuaded management to collaborate in an SAT process to counter the potential move of Xerox's wire harness manufacturing plant to Mexico, which would result in a layoff of 180 workers. Xerox management felt that moving to Mexico was the only way to remain competitive, as relocating outside of the United States would save 30 percent of manufacturing costs per year.[58] The possibility of such a huge layoff, involving more than half of the CMO plant workers, spurred the union to suggest the fairly radical SAT process for discovering cost-saving changes to implement at their plant. Xerox management agreed to this experiment, promising not to relocate their manufacturing department if the $3.2 million they could save by moving was matched in cost savings at the current plant.

Although the SAT process was unproven at that time and could result in radically altered jobs and production processes, the union felt it worth this risk in order to save 180 jobs.

The SAT process at Xerox saved $3.7 million and kept all 180 threatened jobs in Webster through designing and implementing a more effective manufacturing process and purchasing more-efficient new equipment. Soon after the SAT recommendations were implemented, the plant hired a second shift of employees to keep up with new production needs.

In recent years, some manufacturing companies, as well as Maimonides Medical Center,[59] have used the SAT process. More details about how this process works are in chapter 4.

Why Sector Strategies and Study Action Teams Matter in Healthcare

Research by scholars such as the late Clayton Christensen at Harvard University has documented that disruptive changes in healthcare organizations are needed to transform existing systems into those that better serve patients. For Christensen, the new system that is created makes the prior one obsolete.[60] He focuses particularly on the parameters of quality of care, cost control, and treatment outcomes, but does not offer specific suggestions for achieving such significant change.[61] We suggest and will describe the use of sector strategies and Study Action Teams as practical, low-cost methods to foster such disruptive change in healthcare while maximizing resources and limiting risk-taking.

As the U.S. healthcare systems require significant changes to improve the quality of care they provide, improve patient satisfaction, control costs, and respond to new regulations, the need for managed disruptions is becoming increasingly evident: previously dysfunctional systems must change to those that are more staff and patient centered and effective.[62]

Summary

In this chapter, we have discussed the different steps in the evolution of employee participation projects that improve the productivity and effectiveness of their workplaces.

During World War II, the United Auto Workers, led by Walther Reuther, advocated for workers to become involved in discovering methods to accelerate the production of aircraft and tanks for the war effort. This effort was endorsed by President Roosevelt and proved highly successful.

With the Red Scare of the 1950s, the idea of worker and union participation in organizational planning receded, however, as unions began to be viewed with suspicion as Communist inspired. By the 1970s, management scholars had begun to advocate for job enhancement (worker control over the pace of work) and enrichment (employee involvement in ordering materials and planning some aspects of work) to reduce growing worker alienation and absenteeism.

Following a 1972 strike at the Lordstown automotive assembly plant by workers who demanded to play a part in decision making there, the quality of employees' work lives became a critical part of labor negotiations, in addition to strategic discussions about wages and benefits. Shortly afterward, Irving Bluestone organized a QWL initiative at an automotive plant in Tarrytown, New York. Early QWL programs included workers in problem-solving teams that aimed to find solutions to production process problems. At Tarrytown, these teams were quite successful in improving car quality and, as employees felt productively engaged, absenteeism was significantly reduced. During the 1970s and '80s, hundreds of organizations adopted QWL activities. These resembled the QC activities adopted in Japan but included labor unions in overseeing the selection of team members, choosing work areas to focus on, and training teams. QWL activities also focused on improving processes central to the overall organizational strategy, which QC circles often did not.

Over the following decade, several manufacturers adopted the Xerox Corporation's strategy of creating LMPs, which organized improvement activities within structured agreements between employees and administrators. Such Partnerships were based on negotiated agreements listing mutual goals, ground rules, staff assignments, and bud gets. In 1997, Kaiser Permanente developed the first healthcare LMP. Shortly after, Maimonides Hospital and the Los Angeles County Department of Health Services created LMPs, which (1) used sector strategies (at DHS) to adopt Patient Centered Medical Homes for its hospitals and clinics and (2) developed Study Action Teams (Maimonides) to successfully redesign their Hospital Cleanliness system.

CHAPTER 2

European Employee Involvement Practices

> If you want to go fast, go alone. If you want to go far, go together.
>
> —*African proverb*

The role of unions and the role of governmental involvement with labor differ significantly in Scandinavia and elsewhere in Europe from those in the United States. However, a number of successful European practices for employee participation can be used for collaborative healthcare restructuring in the United States. For this reason, we examine in this chapter the most relevant employee participation practices that can be adapted for American healthcare and other organizations.

Workers have had a role in making decisions, sharing responsibility, and at times redesigning work systems in Scandinavian workplaces since the nineteenth century.[63] Collaborative practices have gradually influenced and spread throughout Europe, particularly since World War II, when Scandinavian governments, employers' associations, and trade unions began funding research to increase worker decision making on the shop floor and to make work more meaningful for frontline staff. The term used in Europe for worker participation activities is *industrial democracy.*[64] Within the framework of industrial democracy, all social partners (workers, management, and government) work together toward shared goals that benefit the national economy, local communities, and workers. The workplace becomes, in the minds of these social partners, a locus in which democratic principles are practiced, usually through shared decision making.[65]

The four main goals of industrial democracy as practiced in Scandinavia are as follows:

- Most important, expansion of opportunities for workers to directly participate in deciding about their working conditions.
- The second goal, adopted since the 1980s, has been to use worker participation projects to improve the productivity of Scandinavian companies[66] and of their national economies.
- The third goal, which emerged initially in Norway, views worker participation activities as critical for providing workers with the tools to engage more actively in civic affairs. Workers who have had leadership opportunities, who have learned how to problem-solve and to resolve conflicting viewpoints about work system issues, participate more actively in local civic organizations. The Norwegians, sensitized to how easily fascism spread in the

1940s among disenfranchised, alienated workers in Germany, have viewed this outcome as crucial in order to sustain their active democracy.

- A fourth goal in Denmark and Sweden has been to reduce staff turnover and absenteeism, each a significant societal problem.

In Germany, worker participation initiatives focus on including frontline staff in corporate decision making, as a result of legislation[67] requiring most organizations to have worker representatives on boards of directors. In Norway, Denmark, and Sweden, increasing organizational productivity was not the initial goal of industrial democracy activities.[68] Instead, they sought to allow workers a voice in matters concerning their workplace and its functioning. Yet all social partners understood that loss of productive capacity and earnings was not an acceptable outcome for their nations' economies.[69]

Four Key Practices of Industrial Democracy That Can be Adapted to an American Setting

Self-Managing Work Groups

In the last chapter, we described unit-based teams tasked with solving problems about production, patient care, or other job-centered matters in some American industries. U.S. teams most often contain a management representative. In contrast, self-managing groups, pioneered in Great Britain, give workers the responsibility and authority to organize their own work without the need for a supervisor or manager. This system initially emerged from the work of Eric Trist and Fred Emery, social scientists at the Tavistock Institute in the United Kingdom. The Tavistock Institute is known for its extensive research on new work systems, on labor relations, and on developing effective leaders. Another Tavistock Institute division studies the application of psychoanalytic understandings of group processes to consultations with industry and to issues confronting the larger society.

Trist and Emery discovered the potential of self-managing work groups while conducting research for the British coal industry. England had nationalized its coal mines following World War II to fuel postwar reconstruction. As coal was a key power source, the British economy depended on its being plentiful and inexpensive. There were extensive labor disputes and stoppages involving the coal mines during the 1940s, however, and absentee rates exceeded 20 percent in many mines during this period. The postwar decision to nationalize the industry was motivated by the government's desire to resolve these issues.[70] Continued absenteeism, however, motivated coal industry executives to hire Trist and Emery to analyze what would contribute to better working conditions, improved labor relations, and increased productivity in the mines. They were also interested in learning why certain coal mines were highly productive while others were not.

Observing operations and talking to miners, owners, union leaders, and managers at both low-and high-performing coal mines, Trist and Emery discovered that in the productive mines, the miners had organized themselves into self-managing work groups. This arrangement enabled workers to be much more efficient and effective. They took owner ship of their equipment, discovered better ways to use available technologies, created an ongoing schedule for maintenance and repair of equipment, and took the initiative to communicate between shifts. They ordered the tools and supplies that they needed, scheduled timely preventive maintenance on equipment, and organized a vacation schedule. These miners made sure that everyone in their work group had sufficient time to master the skills needed to operate and maintain all pieces of equipment. Creating multiskilled workers enabled the miners to switch easily from one operation to another. Morale increased among workers using this method, reducing both turnover and absenteeism.[71] On the other hand, in coal mines with low productivity and high absenteeism, researchers observed that miners had traditional discrete jobs with little opportunity to make decisions or switch operations when needed. Once Trist and Emery shared their findings, many mines in the UK shifted their production process to self-managing teams.

Because of the close relationship between the Tavistock Institute researchers and workplace researchers in Norway, Sweden, and Denmark, several self-managing work group projects started in Scandinavia once reports of the experience in the British coal mines were shared internationally.[72]

As described in chapter 1, the environmental services workers at Maimonides Medical Center in Brooklyn shifted to self-managing work groups after the Study Action Team completed its work. Similar work groups were developed at the Hathaway shirt company to implement the new production process that helped keep the plant open. These examples demonstrate the usefulness of self-managing work groups in an American setting.

While most employee participation teams in the United States are not self-managing, accumulating evidence suggests that this strategy is well worth considering here. The practice has not been widely adopted in the United States largely due to the fact that most managers do not learn about it in business schools and are unsure as to its implementation. Unions as well tend to be unfamiliar with this approach.

Socio-Technical Systems Approaches to Work Organizations

The second significant approach emerging from the European experience has been their focus on optimizing *socio-technical systems* (STS).[73] After observing workers in industries who were organized into self-managing work groups, Trist and Emery realized that these workers were optimizing their social organization, their use of technology, *and* the interfaces between the two. Based on these observations, the researchers developed a new theory of organizational design, known as *socio-technical system design*.[74] This approach to creating effective organizations recognizes the interrelatedness of the social dimension of work (whether employees' assignments, for example, are collaborative or occur in isolation, and how they are treated) and the technical systems utilized in their workplaces. "Technical" here encompasses more than just equipment; it refers to both work tools and work processes. The theory emphasizes the importance of finding a better fit between how one works and how one uses available technologies. After their coal mining project, Trist and others at the Tavistock Institute focused on understanding what contributes to an effective "socio-technical system design."[75]

Trist and Emery's pioneering work on socio-technical systems in the UK led to several national projects in Norway and Sweden. One important socio-technical project involved a collaboration between the Swedish National Institute for Working Life, the Volvo Car Group, and the union representing Swedish autoworkers. By the early 1970s, Volvo senior management had decided that they needed to expand their manufacturing capacity in Sweden to produce more cars while simultaneously improving their employees' quality of work life. As in the UK and the United States, absenteeism and staff turnover had become a problem due to workers' alienation from routinized, assembly-line work systems.[76] Planners hoped that by carefully designing new plants in ways that improved the quality of employees' work lives, they could maintain, if not improve, quality standards while reducing absenteeism and employee turnover. The company and union had previously failed to improve these via job enrichment and job enhancement strategies such as making jobs more interesting by rotating workers to different assignments or by adding new responsibilities.[77] These approaches only modified existing production processes without significantly improving them through incorporating workers' ideas and observations.[78]

Ultimately, Volvo senior management and trade union leaders decided upon a more comprehensive systemic change. Pehr G. Gyllenhammar, then president of the Volvo Group and a progressive manager who respected the importance of frontline staff, articulated the challenge that both management and labor faced: "We need to create an environment that will give satisfaction to the employees in their daily tasks. Due to the advanced economic and social structure of Swedish society, we have encountered earlier than most countries new problems in the organization of jobs and the working environment." Facing these problems, he contended, "could well lead to an improvement in competitive ability."[79]

Under Gyllenhammar's leadership and with the full involvement of various Swedish trade union leaders, a new assembly plant in Kalmar, Sweden, was designed using a socio-technical analysis to create new production processes. The design was intended to maximize available technologies for assembling high-quality cars while creating a new work system to provide greater decision-making responsibilities for workers. To apply the socio-technical approach, an Action Committee was formed with an equal number of labor and management members to design the new Kalmar plant. The Action Committee studied other car assembly plant production processes and the technologies they used. The committee then designed the new plant so that groups of employees assembled sections of a car together, instead of having each worker standing at separate workstations, toiling at a repetitive job for 8 to 10 hours each day. The new work groups that were created stayed with the car until they completed all their operations, which usually took 45 minutes to an hour. The car chassis then moved to the next work group, who together assembled the next section of the car. Kalmar began producing cars with this process in 1974.

By the early 1980s, Volvo decided to increase its manufacturing capacity even further. Building on the success of the Kalmar plant in terms of quality and number of cars produced, a second assembly plant design process was initiated with full trade union involvement. The Action Committee for the Uddevalla assembly plant developed an even more radical production process than at Kalmar. In keeping with socio-technical system design practices, this second plant was designed so that work teams of nine individuals had the responsibility for together assembling an entire car. Modern technology was installed to make it easier to weld and assemble each car section. Special carriers were designed so that workers could swivel and turn the entire car, enabling easy access to every area. Working in self-managing groups, employees could determine the rotation of jobs, the pacing of their work throughout the day, and the schedule of workers and training needed. This new process enabled the frontline staff teams to identify production design problems immediately, as they oversaw the entirety of the production process and could identify problems as they occurred. Workers at both the Kalmar and Uddevalla assembly plants received training so that they could perform all assembly jobs in their work group. At the Uddevalla plant, workers could easily observe the fruits of their labor, and they developed a sense of owner ship and gratification from assembling an entire car.[80]

The quality and productivity of the Uddevalla and Kalmar plants were equal to, if not better than, those at other Volvo assembly plants,[81] and absenteeism and employee turnover decreased radically at both plants as well.[82] Chapter 8 presents more details about establishing such new systems.

Employee-Driven Innovations

Scandinavian countries have continued to explore ways for frontline staff to improve the effectiveness of their organizations. In recent years, both union leaders and managers observed that innovative ideas were often sparked by the need to work around day-to-day problems on the job[83] or by employees observing that some work processes or equipment consistently caused problems. The Danish LO (Confederation of Trade Unions) initiated *Employee-Driven Innovation* (EDI) projects in 2007 to expand opportunities for frontline staff to create new services or products. In Denmark, EDI activities primarily focused on increasing innovations in their healthcare systems. These are discussed shortly. Other European countries that adopted the EDI approach have focused on the technology and manufacturing sectors.[84]

Like the United States and other countries, Denmark needs to control costs so that healthcare is affordable. Although the Danish national health system provides all citizens with free healthcare, the government has needed to find alternatives to raising taxes to pay for healthcare services. As in the United States, this has become an increasing challenge as citizens live longer and tend to require more medical and home care services as they age. With funds from regional health departments, private foundations, and the Danish Confederation of Trade Unions, hospital and regional health departments have hired staff to identify workers with fresh ideas for improving patient care while also controlling costs. Projects they have developed include discovering newer, more cost-effective technologies and developing new strategies for providing better home-and community-based care.

EDI staff help frontline workers to frame and develop their new concepts for particular services or potential medical devices. Once such a concept is developed, the frontline employee (doctor, lab technician, or ward clerk) is connected with an expert to help refine the idea, and then to develop a prototype for the new device or conduct a pi lot new service. This expert also helps the employee to develop a business plan for financing the implementation of the concept. At Aalborg University Hospital, for example, the Idéklinikken ("Ideas Clinic") serves as a healthcare service incubator[85] providing time and space for frontline staff to develop their ideas for improving services.

"Many times, frontline staff have great ideas but don't have the ability or time to continue to refine their ideas—turning ideas into real products or service changes," commented Kristine Rasmussen, the Idéklinikken's project manager, during a November 2015 interview.[86] Nurses and physicians are the most common initiators, but any healthcare practitioner can propose a product, a piece of equipment, or an idea for changing a hospital's delivery system or regional health department service.

EDI activities represent a major shift in emphasis from the common practices of employee participation/industrial democracy in Europe. In Denmark, the basic emphasis of EDI activities has been on creating new devices to help patients, particularly aging individuals, have a better quality of life, or creating new processes to improve clinical outcomes. Developing a new product to generate funds for regional health systems is also encouraged.[87] The income from developing a new device is jointly shared by the inventor, EDI, or a particular hospital or health department.

Some products and services created from Danish EDI projects include a mobile app to help adolescents control their diabetes, new home-monitoring equipment for cardiac patients, a pacifier for premature infants to provide them with oxygen while in the intensive care unit, stretch sensors to control for excessive load to an injured foot, a method for improved patient medication management, a new process to connect the physically disabled to community services, and a redesigning of emergency room departments to keep patients comfortable and informed of the status of their care while being treated.

In addition to supporting the development of specific worker-identified projects, beginning in 2007 the Danish LO established the Employee Driven Innovation

Network (EDIN) to enable scholars, consultants, practitioners, funders, product developers, and graduate students throughout Europe to share research findings and develop methods to accelerate the spread of EDI practices. This network has used its funding to assist frontline staff in refining their suggestions for new products and services.

EDI activities have greatly helped Scandinavian countries, enabling them to stretch their limited resources to continue providing all citizens with comprehensive health services at affordable costs. EDI projects have created more meaningful jobs for workers as their ideas are put into practice: "ideas for new products and services and more meaningful work that no one would have thought about if it weren't for the EDI process,"[88] stated Kjeld Lisby, head of innovation at Aalborg University Hospital.

Organizations in the United States that are beginning to use this model are described in chapter 7.

Participatory Action Research

Industrial democracy researchers in Scandinavia and the UK rely on a dynamic research method known as *participatory action research* (PAR). PAR is a tool that supports frontline staff participation by offering practitioners (frontline staff and administrators) the opportunity to work alongside researchers to define questions relevant to their work and to develop methods of documenting outcomes of their projects.

Involvement in deciding which information to obtain and then in actively collecting those data tends to strengthen the commitment of frontline staff to implementing the solutions their research reveals. This method, along with their inclusion in the overall project execution, fosters the owner ship of frontline staff at all stages of the change process.

One of the first to use the PAR approach was the activist Paulo Freire, who employed this methodology in Brazil to encourage deprived communities to research, analyze, and document the structural basis for their lack of resources.[89] Their analysis found persuasive approaches for rectifying the inequitable allocation of resources and was greatly empowering. From these community roots, PAR has developed into an important research method for all types of organizations, from grassroots community groups to medical centers.

PAR differs from traditional research in three ways. First, its goal is to assist in efforts at change within a community or organization, so it is driven by the needs and concerns of members of that group. The goal of traditional research, on the other hand, is to conduct robust, disciplined studies controlling critical variables in order to identify specific causes that result in statistically significant outcomes. Such research aims to discover answers to particular questions of scientific relevance, but it is not focused on implementation or on the needs of a particular organization or community.

Second, PAR projects use a variety of approaches: collecting both qualitative and quantitative data using questionnaires, surveys, focus groups, observation teams, document analysis, etc. Traditional research methodology does not usually include constituents because of concerns about biasing the results, but the variety of tools used in a PAR process affords the opportunity to cross-check and validate findings.

Third, researchers and frontline staff work together to determine how best to share results and lessons learned so that the data gathered can lead to action.[90] With this co-generative research method, an organization creates a comprehensive process to document and analyze current systems and practices, as well as discover information that can lead to the development of new breakthroughs. The process of bringing together researchers and frontline staff affords each group a broader understanding of the others' concerns.[91]

Summary

Discovering ways to sustain and deepen worker participation has been a core focus of numerous workplaces and research organizations in Scandinavia and England since World War II. In Scandinavia, these activities were initially created to increase decision making for workers, to make work more meaningful, to reinforce democratic principles of engagement and participation, and to create labor peace. Gradually the focus of industrial democracy shifted to initiatives to improve the productivity and effectiveness of organizations, to control costs, and to respond to such labor issues as increased absenteeism and staff turnover.

The tools of self-managing work groups, of socio-technical systems design, of Employee-Driven Innovation, and of participatory action research have demonstrated value and are beginning to be employed in the United States, where they can be easily applied to healthcare Labor-Management Partnerships.[92] In addition, the increased participation of workers in civic affairs, resulting from the skills and confidence that such partnerships engender, has been a critical outcome of industrial democracy in Scandinavia.[93] This has great relevance to the United States, where, for example, only 61 percent of voters participated in the electoral process in the 2016 national elections, and where few citizens involve themselves in local or national civic organizations.[94] Details and data about the relationship between workplace and civic participation are presented in chapter 8.

PART TWO

Best Practices

CHAPTER 3

Core Practices of Successful Labor-Management Partnerships

> The current system cannot do the job. Trying harder will not work. Changing systems of care will.
>
> *—Institute of Medicine and the Committee on Quality of Health Care in America*

Over the past 30 years, Labor-Management Partnerships have increased frontline staff participation in decision making within manufacturing, technology firms, federal and state governments, school systems, and healthcare organizations. These joint activities have improved the quality of services and products and contributed to considerable cost reductions in the organizations that have adopted them. As already noted, after creating a comprehensive Labor-Management Partnership, Xerox reduced its manufacturing costs by over 30 percent; in healthcare, Maimonides Medical Center dramatically increased safety by reducing patient falls and hospital-acquired infections by 50 percent and improved overall patient satisfaction with hospital cleanliness by over 75 percent, with a cost savings of 45 percent in supplies.[95]

Current research on best practices of Labor-Management Partnerships conducted by American and European scholars, including the first author,[96] and advice garnered from many practitioners of this method suggests that seven LMP core practices lead to successful outcomes:

(1) Hiring an initial consultant familiar with the most effective methods for enlisting frontline staff and management involvement in Partnership activities.

(2) Developing extensive educational activities for frontline staff and senior leaders so they can understand why changes are needed and how productive change can occur.

(3) Creating a social contract between labor and management that spells out clear ground rules; a defined structure for joint work and decision-making processes; and specific, mutually advantageous goals. When possible, the contract should include an employment security clause.

(4) Developing internal consultants and coaches to support problem-solving work groups and teams.

(5) Improving overall labor relations to encourage employees to work with management, contributing their ideas and advice.

(6) Using sector strategies to identify known ways of achieving successful change.

(7) Creating an effective process for documenting results.

Not every healthcare Labor-Management Partnership initiative focuses on all core practices at once. However, the core practices presented in this chapter serve as a basic roadmap for labor and management leaders in healthcare systems or in other organizations seeking to develop or deepen joint activities.

We illustrate these core practices through two case studies of developing Labor-Management Partnerships in healthcare organizations. The first case study concerns the development of a Labor-Management Partnership at Maimonides Medical Center, a stand-alone hospital offering extensive outpatient services and actively interfacing with community groups. The second case study involves the Labor Management Partnership at the Los Angeles County Department of Health Services (LA-DHS), the second-largest public health system in the United States, encompassing four major hospitals and 17 ambulatory care facilities.

As W. Edwards Deming, the quality control guru in the 1980s, stated, there is "no instant pudding for transforming organizations—it is a marathon, not a sprint."[97]

We have tried to capture enough basic details from each case to illustrate the nature of these "marathons" and to describe how these core activities supported Partnership work. We indicate the key roles that collaborative leaders have played in implementing these core practices.

Case Study 1: Maimonides Medical Center

Over 100 years old, Maimonides Medical Center is a respected treatment facility and academic medical center in Brooklyn, New York. Serving people of all faiths and backgrounds from the borough's extremely diverse population, Maimonides Medical Center has 705 inpatient beds and more than 70 primary care and subspecialty programs. Each year it records more than 80,000 emergency room visits, 210,000 ambulatory care visits, and 6,700 infant deliveries. As such, it is one of the busiest medical centers in New York State. It also trains more than 400 medical and surgical residents annually.

Maimonides started its Labor-Management Partnership process (referred to as their "Strategic Alliance") in 1997. The Alliance reflected the shared vision of Executive Vice President Pam Brier and the late John Reid, then executive vice president of Service

Employees International Union (SEIU) Local 1199, to establish a joint working process for labor and management to meet the challenges of the rapidly changing healthcare environment. The 1994 collective bargaining agreement between SEIU 1199 and the League of Voluntary Hospitals and Homes of New York, to which Maimonides belongs, articulated the importance of such joint work to improve patient care in League hospitals and nursing homes. This historic agreement did not, however, detail which activities would be most helpful, nor how to implement them.

The success of the eventually robust Strategic Alliance at Maimonides Medical Center to a large extent reflects the collaborative leadership[98] of Brier, Reid, and eventually Bruce Richard, former executive vice president of SEIU 1199, and the extremely motivated frontline staff who contributed to redesigning work processes in many areas of the hospital.

Pam Brier, a progressive healthcare administrator who worked for many years in New York City hospitals, was a pro-worker community activist who was passionate about improving patient care. She teamed up with John Reid a little over a year after she became executive vice president of Maimonides in 1995. Brier eventually became the president and CEO of Maimonides in 2003. For years she had wanted to find ways to improve the working relationship between labor and management. Reid was a veteran union leader, deeply involved in civil rights issues, who was already beginning to move SEIU 1199 away from being a traditional union to one proactive about the changes taking place in healthcare systems. Later, Bruce Richard, another SEIU 1199 executive VP, assumed Reid's role as the key union leader working with Brier at Maimonides. Richard, a community organizer and social justice advocate, brought his own experience working as a meter collector in New York, where he had experimented with implementing self-managing work teams.[99]

The Affordable Care Act of 2010, which placed quality control demands on hospitals and provided health insurance for close to 20 million Americans, had not yet been conceived in 1997. It was nonetheless clear to Brier and Reid that healthcare delivery systems in Brooklyn and elsewhere in New York State needed to radically improve their quality of and access to care, while at the same time controlling costs. Brier and Reid shared the goal of using a worker participation process to address these issues within the Medical Center while creating meaningful work for frontline staff.

As there were then very few Labor-Management Partnership models in healthcare organizations, Brier and Reid hired Lazes as a consultant to advise them about initiating their Strategic Alliance process (Core Practice 1). He suggested that they visit the Saturn Corporation for a close-up view of an existing, highly successful Labor-Management Partnership process. Lazes was familiar with the Saturn Partnership, having served as an early consultant to their process. The

Saturn trip provided a valuable experiential education (Core Practice 2) for key union and management leaders from Maimonides in what a Labor-Management Partnership (LMP) process could achieve and in how it worked.

Reid and Brier quickly formed a delegation of hospital union and management leaders to meet with personnel in corresponding positions and with frontline staff at Saturn's manufacturing plant in Spring Hill, Tennessee. They hoped to learn about how the LMP process at Saturn had been developed, how its employees had experienced its growth, and how management and labor had worked out their differences. From this site visit, they learned firsthand the importance of the key practices described in this chapter. Most impressive, according to Brier and Reid, was their observation of the extensive research undertaken by the workforce, union leaders, and plant management before constructing the factory (Core Practice 2), in order to learn the most up-to-date sector strategies (Core Practice 6) for automobile manufacturing. A labor-management task force at Saturn ("the Committee of 99")[100] had spent a year amassing considerable data about what was working and what was not for their parent company, General Motors, and their competitors, and had investigated cost controls with an eye toward producing an affordable, attractive compact car to compete with popular Japanese models.

Maimonides representatives were also impressed by the details incorporated into Saturn's social contract (Core Practice 3). This document, which they closely examined, set ground rules from which a culture of collaboration took shape and continued to grow, as well as a clear process for problem identification, problem solving, and decision making. At Saturn, management and the union agreed to a decision-making process in which the union would be a full partner in all decisions.

This educational site visit provided an experience that was crucial for convincing union leaders, as well as middle-level and senior managers at Maimonides, of the value of initiating an LMP for their hospital. Upon returning to Maimonides, union and management leaders established a two-hour educational workshop for all employees. The goal was to share with all staff the challenges facing Maimonides and other hospitals in New York City (Core Practice 2). Maimonides was facing changes in state and federal reimbursements, particularly payments for Medicare patients, that now tied levels of reimbursement to treatment quality and patient satisfaction scores. There was also the possibility that for-profit hospitals might be entering the New York healthcare market as competitors for patients.

In order to model a joint process for Partnership at Maimonides, these and subsequent educational workshops were conducted by a joint team comprising a union leader and a manager. For frontline staff, this collaborative leadership approach demonstrated a radical change in the hospital's practices. Collaborative leadership is a style of organizational management that fosters the roles of labor and management as co-leaders who encourage frontline line staff to share their knowledge and expertise about problems in their institution. Collaborative leaders enable staff to identify and solve problems that they experience firsthand, and to implement their solutions. Such an approach encourages staff to eventually become leaders in their organization.

The co-facilitated workshops also conveyed to frontline staff that the unions at Maimonides SEIU 1199 and the New York State Nurses Association [NYSNA])[101] were active partners in these activities. Beyond sharing information about the changing healthcare landscape in New York City, the workshops solicited suggestions from frontline staff about patient care problems that required resolution. Attending physicians, department chairs, residents, and interns went to these participatory educational workshops along with nurses, social workers, environmental service employees, security guards, dieticians, pharmacists, food service workers, and receptionists.

A few SEIU 1199 and NYSNA shop stewards initially resisted attending the workshops, convinced that their unions would essentially be colluding with management, whose job it was to solve patient care issues, not theirs. Reid, however, used one-on-one meetings with these individuals to explain how true collaborative Partnership activities, such as the one at Saturn, had actually increased union membership and member involvement in union activities. It had also given workers a voice in daily decision making about their jobs and the equipment they used. Several managers similarly did not accept the need to consult frontline staff about ways to improve patient care, or to decide on the purchasing of equipment or supplies. In similar one-on-one sessions with these managers, Brier found that a successful strategy was to encourage hesitant managers to begin with a low-risk project that might help them learn through experience the specific benefits of frontline staff participation.

Having completed the initial educational and focus groups, Brier and Reid organized a daylong retreat with key management, union leaders, and frontline staff. This highly interactive work session focused on clarifying why and how a Labor-Management Partnership would be helpful for Maimonides, drafting some joint goals for their Strategic Alliance process, and identifying some initial joint activities. I (Lazes) facilitated the work session, which included breakout meetings for discussions with small groups of frontline staff. Throughout the day, Reid, Brier, and I encouraged all participants to express their concerns about the Partnership process and suggested areas in the hospital that could benefit from the initial Partnership work groups.

This retreat created an opportunity for frontline staff, from environmental services employees to attending physicians, to comfortably contribute their ideas and concerns. For most frontline staff, inclusion in a conversation with the president of the hospital and several medical department chairs was an uncommon experience. To create a respectful and welcoming setting, the retreat had an agenda based on understanding the concerns of all stakeholders, not just those of senior management. This helped to create a more level playing field so that all participants gained comfort in expressing their viewpoints without fear of criticism. Participants were encouraged to contribute to large and small group work sessions throughout the day.

The agreements reached at the retreat became the heart of the LMP social contract (Core Practice 3). This document included goals for joint work (that is, issues important to Maimonides unions and managers for the Partnership to address), a plan for initial project activities, a bud get for relieving frontline staff of their usual responsibilities to work on problem-solving teams, and the creation of a Labor-Management Strategic Alliance Council as a governance structure that would oversee hospital-wide and unit-level projects. Three new positions for internal consultants (Core Practice 4) were established to support Partnership activities. Finally, an innovative agreement was forged concerning who would decide whether to accept the recommendations of the various problem-solving teams. Such decisions would be arrived at jointly, rather than solely by management, and would be based on the data that the different teams gathered in support of their proposals. It was agreed, too, that administrators would share departmental bud gets and patient care data with frontline staff teams, so that they would have the necessary information to further their work. This social contract also clarified that no employee would lose his or her job as a result of LMP activities.

Membership in the Labor-Management Strategic Alliance Council comprised union and management leaders, as well as frontline employees from the inpatient and outpatient laboratory, and from the Departments of Food and Nutrition, Engineering, Ambulatory Care, Nursing, and Medicine. The hospital's chief medical director, the director of the Emergency Department, the director for labor relations and performance improvement, the chief financial officer, and the president/CEO of Maimonides were also Council members. Additional members were added to the council as work expanded to other departments of the hospital.

Initially, frontline staff participation activities focused on three departments: Radiology, Food and Nutrition, and the inpatient and outpatient laboratory. A hospital-wide committee, the Joint Hiring Committee, was established to develop joint goals for hiring new managers and supervisors. In each department, I provided unit-based teams with conflict-resolution and problem-solving training and taught them how to use workflow diagrams to analyze work roles and processes in underperforming areas. Details of how such unit-based teams accomplished their work appear in chapter 4.

As at Xerox, to support the transformation to a frontline staff-participation culture at Maimonides, Brier and Reid created the position of internal consultants (termed "Developers") to assist and support Partnership work groups (Core Practice 4). These leaders witnessed the need for neutral mentors, working with both labor and management as coaches and educators, during their Saturn visit. Such mentors oversaw the progress of the work groups and ensured that their members received education, training, and support to accomplish their goals. The Developers worked with Maimonides' middle managers and shop stewards to ensure that frontline staff were freed from their normal duties to attend work group meetings and that meeting rooms were available to them. Co-chairs of the committees found the internal consultants' assistance with work group preparation and follow-up assignments quite helpful.[102] Besides assisting individual work groups, the internal consultants ("Developers") met periodically with shop stewards and supervisors to discover new approaches that might help support Strategic Alliance activities and overall labor relations (Core Practice 5).

In these basic ways, internal consultants helped ensure that Partnership activities were well organized and that the various teams focused on the problems they were tasked to solve. This, along with ensuring that teams consulted with any worker whom their recommendations would potentially affect—an important aspect of collaborative leadership—helped most teams to achieve positive results. Having internal consultants has enabled Maimonides, over the years, to broaden and sustain worker participation activities without relying further on my consultations.[103]

At Maimonides, all three Developers (one rank-and-file member of each union[104]) and one manager were paid by the hospital. They were chosen by senior union and management leaders. Selecting employees for this role was based on their ability to work with others, on their communication skills, and on their ability to encourage employees to work together. Their training included education in successful methods for achieving organizational change, effective Labor-Management Partnerships practices, methods to support groups and group leaders, and the use of socio-technical analysis tools to optimize the interface between jobs and various technologies. In addition, they learned methods for developing workflow and cost-benefit analyses, and strategies for unblocking teams when they experienced an impasse.[105] More details about how to unblock groups that are not functioning well are presented in chapter 5.

Cornell University's Healthcare Transformation Project, the Performance Improvement staff of Maimonides, and the SEIU 1199 League Labor-Management Project staff[106] provided the training for the Developers, each of whom was assigned to a specific department.

Notably, several of the original Developers eventually assumed important leadership roles at Maimonides and SEIU 1199 after leaving these internal consultant jobs. Two Developers were appointed to positions in the Labor Relations department—one became its director—and a third Developer was elected a vice president for SEIU 1199. This resulted from their effectiveness in helping frontline staff work together, their ability to get others to work out differences between staff, and their passion to create meaningful work for employees.

Creating a bud get for internal consultants and selecting talented and flexible staff for this role has proved critical at Maimonides, as well as in all of the Labor-Management Partnerships cited in this book. The expectation that effective joint work can occur without supportive infrastructures, including a governance process and internal consultants, is one of the most frequent reasons for the failure of Labor-Management Partnerships to achieve effective organizational change.[107]

The fifth Core Practice cited in almost all Labor-Management Partnership research is the importance of strengthening labor relations so that they are fair and respectful. "Without a positive relationship between frontline staff and management, it is hard, if not impossible, to encourage employees to share their knowledge and skills,"[108] asserted Diane Factor, director of the Worker Education and

Resource Center at LA-DHS/SEIU, whose LMP is discussed shortly.

At Maimonides, although labor relations were reasonably unconflicted from the beginning, their Labor-Management Strategic Alliance Council took specific steps to strengthen it, using a threefold approach. In the departments where Labor-Management Partnership activities were initially focused, the Developers, along with labor relations staff, organized workshops for both management supervisors and shop stewards. These workshops, held during lunch hours (Lunch and Learn Sessions), offered an opportunity to discuss in more detail why changes were needed at Maimonides and to explore ways to practice proactive and positive labor relations. Role-playing exercises eased what had sometimes been an adversarial or distant relationship to become collaborative, problem-solving endeavors.

One example of how this process worked occurred in the Environmental Services Department. An employee on the first shift, an excellent worker with a stellar attendance record for several years, began to experience difficulty getting to work on time for her morning shift. After several warnings and one suspension by her supervisor, the employee was notified that her job was in jeopardy.

Using this situation to practice a problem-solving approach to labor relations, the supervisor and union steward in her department explored, via role playing, ways to inquire about and resolve this problem. Upon meeting with the service worker, they discovered that she had a young daughter who had recently developed asthma. When her child's asthma flared up at night, the worker needed to arrange a babysitter on short notice, and occasionally, when the flare-up was severe, she brought her daughter to the pediatrician the following morning. What would have normally resulted in another suspension for tardiness shifted to *what could be done* to respond to her family situation. After much discussion, a solution emerged: the employee would start her shift an hour later than usual, giving her sufficient time to secure a sitter if her daughter became ill. And if her daughter required medical attention, the employee agreed to immediately call the department to inform them of her situation. This solution was implemented, and tardiness was no longer an issue.

Several other activities have been helpful in improving labor relations at Maimonides. One has been to incorporate information about the Maimonides work culture, emphasizing the importance of frontline staff engagement, into the orientation process for all new employees. Orientation sessions describe specific examples of how labor and management work together at all levels of the organization to improve patient care and job satisfaction. The annual review process for managers, supervisors, and department heads now routinely evaluates their record regarding labor relations and their participation with frontline staff in joint activities. These reflection sessions are also used to explore additional ways for the managers to improve labor relations and worker participation opportunities in their department.

A third important activity for supporting positive labor relations has been the creation of joint hiring committees, one of the first hospital-wide projects. These committees were established in each area of the hospital to strengthen the interview process for new department heads, supervisors, and managers, determining whether a particular candidate fits the Maimonides philosophy and values. Even if a candidate previously worked in an organizational culture similar to that of Maimonides, it is important to assess her or his managerial philosophy to determine whether the candidate would be able to contribute to the hospital's joint work culture. The joint hiring process requires all candidates for management and supervisory positions to be interviewed by both frontline and labor relations staff. Their recommendations on whether or not to hire the candidates are then presented to senior management, who make the final hiring decision. Over the years, senior management has accepted all of the recommendations of the joint hiring committees.

Establishing processes that measure the changes resulting from the Alliance work groups (Core Practice 7) has been pursued rigorously at Maimonides. Their monitoring and documentation process has been a joint effort spearheaded by researchers from Cornell

University's Healthcare Transformation Project[109] and assisted by the three internal Developers and the director of leadership development. Involving Cornell and the Developers has helped ensure timely and organized data collection on each project.

Biannual reviews of Partnership activity outcomes by the Labor-Management Strategic Alliance Council has made it possible to track and analyze factors contributing to project successes and shortcomings (see table 2). Having updates available on the current progress of all teams and committees is particularly important "so that frontline staff can receive information about the successes or shortcomings of their new processes and then make adjustments,"[110] observed Susan Goldberg, director of performance improvement at Maimonides Medical Center.

Case Study 2: Los Angeles County Department of Health Services

The Los Angeles County Department of Health Services (LA-DHS), the second-largest public health system in the United States, includes four hospitals, two large multiservice ambulatory care centers, 17 community health centers, and more than 160 community partner clinics providing primary care. LA-DHS treats 750,000 patients annually, most of whom receive Medicaid or are uninsured, and employs more than 18,460 staff. The unions representing workers at LA-DHS are the Committee of Interns and Residents (CIR); the Union of American Physicians and Dentists (UAPD); the American Federation of State, County and Municipal Employees (AFSCME) 2712 and 3511, which represent social workers and psychologists; and SEIU 721, which represents most other hospital workers, including nurses, lab techs, and coders.

Table2. Summary of Prominent Outcomes of Maimonides' Strategic Alliance Activities

Areas for Improvements	Outcomes
Absenteeism in housekeeping staff	Reduction of absenteeism by 25%.
Equipment and supplies available at the beginning of each shift for environmental service workers	100% of the time as opposed to rarely.
Housekeeping supplies	Reduction of 49% of costs.
Obtaining uncollected bills	Increased 75% of collections.
Medication reconciliation completed	From 35% to 95%.
Patient overall satisfaction scores for the cleanliness of rooms and public areas	From 67 % to 85%.
Patient meals delivered on time	Increased from 68% to 93%.
Productivity of engineering department	Increased efficiencies by 80%.
Reduction in hospital-acquired infections	Reduced by 50%.
Reduction in labor-management arbitrations	Reduced by 100%.
Reduction in grievances	Reduction of 63%.
Reduction in turnaround time to and from ER to radiology department	From 90 minutes to less than 30 minutes.
Reduction in patient falls	Reduced by 50%.
Response time to cardiac monitors	From 2.5–8 minutes to less than 1 minute.

Areas for Improvements	Outcomes
Transport time for patients to and from the ED for x-rays	Reduced by 40%.
Turnaround time of lab results to the ER	From two to three hours to 30 minutes.

The passage and funding of the Affordable Care Act (ACA) in 2010 allowed formerly uninsured Los Angeles residents to purchase care from various county hospitals. Hospital administrators and union officials at LA-DHS realized that they needed to become a provider of choice for patients in order to remain competitive. They recognized that creating better access to care and ensuring better integration of services so that patients routinely received coordinated, respectful treatment, were imperative.

When Dr. Mitchell Katz, an internist, was hired as director of LA-DHS in 2011, he quickly initiated discussions with Bob Schoonover and Gilda Valdez, SEIU 721's president and chief of staff, to explore ways to collaborate on changing their system's structure and culture. Before coming to Los Angeles, Katz was the director of the Public Health Department for San Francisco and the director of outpatient services for San Francisco General Hospital. He had found working with healthcare unions in San Francisco quite productive.

Some LA-DHS senior managers were skeptical, however, about establishing a Partnership process with SEIU and the other unions. Accustomed to top-down initiatives, they had doubts about the capacity of the unions and frontline workers to collaborate productively and efficiently.[111] Similarly, many of SEIU 721's executive board, senior leaders, frontline staff, and shop stewards questioned whether management was serious and committed to a bona fide partnership. In 2007, an early Partnership process established at LA-DHS had suffered from a lack of clear, long-term joint goals, the absence of a mutually acceptable governance and decision-making process, and a failure to free up frontline staff from their daily responsibilities to participate in the various work groups. It had failed dismally.

Acknowledging the skeptics' concerns, Katz, Schoonover, and Valdez decided that they needed a more comprehensive and effective Partnership process. They felt pressured by the new Affordable Care Act regulations about access, quality of care, and patient satisfaction, which threatened the survival of several hospitals in their system.

After meeting a number of times, Schoonover, Valdez, and Katz agreed to establish a new Labor-Management Partnership process based on creating joint goals and structures that would better support and sustain frontline staff participation. These leaders acknowledged that for patients to achieve better access to coordinated care, many frontline staff jobs would need to change, and the culture had to as well: patients needed to be treated with more respect and dignity, which had not always been the case.[112] "A significant paradigm shift was needed—not just minor changes,"[113] commented Valdez. This time, the LA-DHS Partnership process was envisioned by both union and management senior leaders as one that would be forward-thinking and that would incorporate the interests and needs of all stakeholders and employees as well as patients.

Schoonover, Valdez, and Katz decided to model the Partnership process on the core practices established at Maimonides, which by this time had achieved demonstrable success. They agreed to lead these activities jointly, collaborating with each other on all aspects of the Partnership. Because of co-author Lazes' strong relationship with the national SEIU leadership and his involvement at Maimonides, they hired him as the outside consultant to guide the initial phases of the LMP (Core Practice 1). Lazes suggested a one-day retreat for all key stakeholders to begin a new and different Labor-Management Partnership process at LA-DHS. The focus of the retreat was to help labor and management leaders, middle managers, and frontline staff at LA-DHS understand the financial and quality of care requirements now being demanded of the county's healthcare system and begin a process that would identify practical methods for meeting them. Another objective for the daylong work session was to encourage frontline staff and managers to articulate goals that were important to them for the Partnership process to address (Core Practice 3).

Three initial goals for the new Labor-Management Partnership process were important to the unions. The first was to establish an intensive educational process throughout LA-DHS (Core Practice 2) so that all employees could learn about current state and federal mandates to improve patient care and the patient experience.[114] These educational activities, to be conducted primarily by the SEIU 721 leaders, would clarify that the county's healthcare system needed to be restructured to become more patient-centered. This meant that many jobs and services would have to be redesigned. The second goal, articulated by the unions and by all frontline staff at the retreat, was that training be provided so that employees could learn the new skills required for their new jobs and job responsibilities. The third goal for the union was to improve labor-relations practices in the LA-DHS.

For management, major goals for the Partnership consisted of reducing the time it took for patients to register and to see a primary care provider; establishing a system so that patients would be seen by the same primary care provider for each of their visits; and ensuring a speedier process for obtaining appointments, particularly with specialists.

Participants at the retreat identified two additional systemwide goals. The first was to standardize the emergency response codes that notified emergency teams across all LA-DHS hospitals and ambulatory clinics of the need for their immediate assistance. The second was to develop a method to monitor and document Partnership activities (Core Practice 7) across the county health system to determine their impact and to communicate the results of their efforts throughout the system.

Work groups formed to address each of these goals composed of members of the LA-DHS Labor-Management Transformation Council and other frontline staff: nurses, housekeeping staff, nursing assistants, and coders. Each work group formulated a quantifiable goal and an anticipated time frame for when this goal would be achieved (e.g., to reduce clinic waiting time for patients by 40 percent in the next two months). After two meetings following up from the retreat, a full social contract (Core Practice 3) and an agreement to create seven internal consultants (Core Practice 4) were established.

The initial work of the LA-DHS Partnership process included implementing Core Practices 1–4, a start at rectifying historically uneven labor-relations practices (5), using a sector strategy (6), and the creation of processes for monitoring and documentation (7). We focus here on Core Practices 6 and 7 (creating sector strategies and documentation/measurement processes), which this system pursued in depth and as such illustrates particularly well.

As mentioned in chapter 1, employing a strategy of proven use in similar organizations can be extremely helpful when attempting to transform an unproductive work system into one that is more effective.

Research by the Commonwealth Foundation, the Robert Wood Johnson Foundation, the Kaiser Foundation, and other organizations has documented that the Patient-Centered Medical Home care process is a successful structure for improving patient care by creating an integrated healthcare delivery system.[115] As noted, this approach improves overall patient outcomes, enhances the patient experience,[116] and controls healthcare costs. The latter is accomplished through reducing hospitalizations, hospital readmissions, duplicate lab work, and unnecessary radiological studies. Creating a "Medical Home" can achieve a better coordinated care delivery system. This includes such practices as the following:

- Patients seeing the same primary care provider at each appointment.
- Patients receiving active follow-up and education about their diagnoses and treatments so that they can more actively manage their health.
- Patients with chronic conditions such as diabetes, heart disease, hypertension, and asthma being treated based on protocols that emphasize best practices.
- Specialists and primary care providers following well-defined processes for documenting and communicating their findings and recommendations with each other and with behavioral health practitioners. In most Medical Homes, this involves

the use of some type of electronic medical records system to share lab data and test results.

Healthcare systems that employ these methods, such as Kaiser Permanente, also use a reimbursement system that pays for staff time to integrate services and provide educational support for patients. Creating Medical Homes requires a fundamental shift in how care is delivered, and it takes time to implement all aspects of this new system.[117]

A key goal that Katz emphasized when he came to Los Angeles was the importance of creating such Patient-Centered Medical Homes within the countywide system. The challenge for the county has been how to transform their large and fragmented delivery system into a more accessible and better integrated one.

To enable the key unions participating in the Partnership process to understand this approach and to determine how to support it, the union's research department located many articles regarding the use, practices, and outcomes of PCMHs. This research revealed that while Medical Homes are quite successful, implementing them within existing healthcare systems is not easy. The new delivery system required changes in the jobs of frontline staff, from primary care providers (doctors, nurses, nurse practitioners, social workers, pharmacists, etc.) to receptionists and call center staff, in order to succeed. The union learned that frontline staff would generally need to work in teams, rather than as solo practitioners. Despite initial resistance, key union leaders became convinced of the necessity for changing the delivery systems to obtain crucial funding for both hospital and ambulatory care facilities. After several internal meetings, leadership from all unions agreed to support the transformation of LA-DHS facilities into PCMHs. Schoonover assigned Patricia Castillo, an energetic and effective union staffer known for her intense involvement and passion for providing a voice for workers, to work with LA-DHS management on devising effective ways to implement the Medical Home model as well as in the overall Labor-Management Partnership process. Castillo was highly valued for her immense creativity and personal warmth. While mentoring the internal consultants, she established strong personal relationships that were highly motivating and that enabled her to offer crucial suggestions to them without being perceived as critical.[118]

To understand the role of frontline staff in implementing Medical Homes at LA-DHS, it is important to know how the county delivery system functioned beforehand.

At the outset of the LMP's formation, county facilities were far from patient-centered. Patients did not have an assigned primary care provider. When they came for clinic appointments, they were seen by whichever doctor or nurse was available, often someone who was unaware of their medical history. Scheduling of doctors in outpatient services was largely based on the educational needs of interns and residents rather than on patient care considerations. Besides not having a permanent primary care practitioner, patients had difficulty in obtaining appointments and limited access to behavioral health providers and other specialists.

Further, patients were given block appointments—that is, all patients were told to come to the clinic at either 9a.m. or 1p.m. and consequently often spent hours waiting to be seen. This practice produced a large no-show rate.[119] This type of healthcare delivery structure resembles that of other U.S. public health systems, such as those at Cook County Health in Chicago and in parts of the NYC Health + Hospitals system. Thus, at LA-DHS the challenge was not whether the transformation into PMCHs was the right strategy, but rather, how to put this new care model into practice.

Here are examples of how frontline staff contributed to implementing aspects of the Medical Home care delivery system in two LA-DHS ambulatory clinics. Initial efforts in the Hubert Humphrey Comprehensive Health Center involved improving patient access to care: creating an appointment system so that patients could be seen more quickly and reducing the time that patients waited to be seen. The second clinic, the Martin Luther King Jr. Outpatient Center, which had already changed its appointment process, focused on improving clinical outcomes.

Improving Access to Care

Continuous improvement teams (CITs), similar to the unit-based teams established in the Kaiser Permanente Partnership process, were already slowly being implemented in several LA-DHS facilities at about the time that Katz and Schoonover established the new Partnership process. After creating Medical Homes became a central goal, more teams were established to get them up and running in ambulatory care clinics throughout the system.

At the Hubert Humphrey Comprehensive Health Center in South Los Angeles, for example, one team, aimed at improving the method of scheduling primary care physician and specialist appointments, was composed of registration staff, a primary care practitioner, staff from the LA-DHS call center who arranged patient appointments, and the manager responsible for registration and preregistration activities. A second CIT team, with similar employee composition, worked on lowering clinic wait times. The teams studied different ways to schedule nurse and physician visits and researched more efficient methods for obtaining patients' insurance information before they arrived for their appointments. Each CIT analyzed ways to reduce no-show appointments.

Both CITs created flow charts to map current patient wait times for appointments and their actual wait times at the facility itself. After analyzing these charts, consulting co-workers, and speaking with patients about what would help them, the teams posed solutions for removing bottlenecks and for streamlining the scheduling, intake, and preregistration processes.

Some of the results that CITs achieved at the Humphrey Health Center were as follows:

- All patients now receive individual appointment times, rather than a block appointment.
- All patients are now assigned a care team.
- A new preregistration process was established for all Humphrey patients, ascertaining their insurance coverage and obtaining advance information needed for the appointment, which increased preregistration from 28 percent to 76 percent.
- Wait time to see a primary care provider, once a patient arrived at the clinic, was reduced from 23 minutes to 3 minutes.

CIT work at the Humphrey Health Center continues to focus on these issues. Such an ongoing process is essential to ensure that the new process becomes fully implemented and functions optimally.[120]

"The engagement of frontline staff in creating more access to care, reduced wait times, and coordinated care has been significant. The fact that workers had a voice in planning the new systems resulted in their endorsing the changes in staff jobs that came along with the new scheduling methods. Staff feel better about working here now,"[121] observed Nicole Moore, director of CITs at LA-DHS.

Implementing Medical Homes and Improving Patient Care Outcomes

The Martin Luther King Jr. Outpatient Center in South Los Angeles, another county facility, transitioned in 2007 from being a small inpatient hospital to a multiservice outpatient center offering a full spectrum of primary care and specialty services. With this transition came individualized appointment systems for patients for primary care and specialty services, and streamlined processes guaranteeing timely patient appointments. Now part of the new Partnership process, King used its continuous improvement teams primarily to convert their outpatient facility into several high-functioning Patient-Centered Medical Homes and to improve clinical outcomes.

In early 2012, the King Center began this process. There are now four King Medical Homes serving adults, children, and patients with HIV diagnoses. If patients come to King who are not already assigned to a specific Medical Home, they are first seen by the Urgent Care Center and then referred for continued care in a particular Medical Home unit.

To improve patient care in the new structures, Partnership action teams are encouraged to work on any clinical problem of importance to their group, but they largely tend to focus on meeting specific patient care outcomes that will help their center secure state and federal funds. This is important financially, as patient care outcomes are tracked by California's Department of Public Health, which sets reimbursements based on outcomes classified as "prime measures."[122] Prime measures include educating diabetic and chronic pain patients about managing their conditions, ensuring that patients obtain a yearly flu shot, increasing screenings for breast and cervical cancer, improving medication reconciliation after each visit to avoid complications caused by drug interactions, and helping patients control their blood pressure. Many King teams have focused on improving outcomes of these measures. These work groups have functioned much as did the ones at Humphrey: following a disciplined process of analyzing current practices, reviewing relevant articles about best practices, consulting with co-workers and patients, and then establishing trial runs of the newly devised processes.

Recent outcomes of these clinical Partnership teams at the King health center have included the following:

Breast cancer screening: Increased by 31 percent

Colorectal cancer screening: Increased from 35 to 72 percent

Controlling blood pressure: Decreased the number of patients with uncontrolled blood pressure by 29 percent

Clinical depression: Screening increased by 10 percent

Diabetic education for patients: Increased by 96 percent (from 31 to 75 percent)

Flu vaccines: Increased the number of flu vaccines by 757 percent from 54 to 409 given through February 2019

Flu shots for patients (Women's Clinic): Increased by 359 percent

No-shows in Gastroenterology: Decreased from 34 to 18.5 percent

Patient satisfaction scores for the health center: Now are over 91 percent

Skin cancer—compliance with treatment protocols: Increased to 96 percent[123]

Creating the structure of Patient-Centered Medical Homes and developing ways to improve clinical outcomes at LA-DHS has been, of necessity, a gradual process. "Although this new care model has not been fully implemented within all county facilities, over 350,000 patients are now empaneled [e.g., assigned to a specific PCMH]. What is proving to be most important is that patients are getting more access to care and feeling better about the care that they are receiving,"[124] observed Dr. David Campa, director of the Primary Care/Ambulatory Care Network, about the process. He added that "if we hadn't started this process with a clear model [the Patient-Centered Medical Home], it would have taken much longer and we would still be experimenting with different approaches."[125]

One important investment that has enhanced the King Center patient experience has been the hiring of community health workers to follow up with patients after their appointments. Community workers ensure that patients understand and follow care recommendations prescribed by patients' primary care teams. They help their patients practice self-care measures and encourage them to follow recommended dietary changes. They also gauge medication compliance. Hiring these new frontline staff, plus new processes established to better coordinate primary care and behavioral health providers, has substantially improved patients' experience at King.[126]

Creating an Effective Process to Document Results

Establishing procedures for documenting the work teams' recommendations and outcomes (Core Practice 7) has presented a challenge within this large system. Typically, work group members have wanted to focus on implementing their newly created solutions and have resented somewhat the time it takes to document each specific intervention and its outcome. "Why document what we are doing, when we can see for ourselves that it works?" has been a sentiment commonly voiced by some labor and management leaders and frontline staff.

It is difficult enough to free frontline staff from their regular duties to analyze and formulate solutions to institutional problems. Making the time for them to document results can be very difficult to justify in institutions with tight bud gets. Yet, ensuring that there is a process to measure the outcomes of problem-solving teams at LA-DHS has been essential in order to gauge whether or not their interventions are achieving the intended results. Further, timely documentation shared with staff (as cited previously) enables them to evaluate how their interventions are working and to adjust them accordingly. Finally, these data are important to justify the investment in Partnership activities to management and to union leaders.[127]

To address this challenge, the Continuous Improvement Team Oversight Committee, established to support and monitor team activities, was assigned the responsibility of ensuring that documentation was being accomplished in each setting. The local union assigned Patricia Castillo to work with Nicole Moore, chair of the CIT Oversight Committee, to make sure that documentation processes were practical and could be easily implemented. In addition, senior management and union leaders on the Labor-Management Transformation Council formally agreed that data collected from Partnership activities would not be used to discipline frontline staff if their goals were not met, but rather would be used to identify continued areas for improvement. This ground rule was particularly important for frontline staff. "We weren't sure how the results of our team would eventually be used. We initially feared that this information might be used to discipline us. After several months of measuring outcomes of our work, though, we saw that this data was being used only to identify areas of work where improvements continued to be needed. Making sure that patient feedback and care improvement practices are not used as a disciplinary tool has been really important so staff don't resist getting feedback about their team's work,"[128] commented Wilson Mendez, a physical therapist and a Healthcare Transformation Advocate, at the King Outpatient Center. Mendez, an energetic man with gentle yet persuasive charisma, assisted numerous teams in their work. He was known to possess a special skill for helping his teams stay focused at solving the clinical problems they had chosen to address. In recognition of his work, Mendez is currently being considered for membership on the County's Committee to Oversee Partnership Activities.

Besides overseeing the overall documentation process, the Continuous Improvement Oversight Committee captured how some of the work groups functioned by videotaping their team meetings and presentations. These videotapes provide useful qualitative data to analyze CIT leadership approaches and member participation. They also help to identify teams that might need assistance in working together or in choosing more realistic projects. To a large extent, the Healthcare Transformation Advocates (internal consultants) have become central to mining this information to determine which of their assigned groups need assistance.

Summary

The case studies of Maimonides and LA-DHS in this chapter illustrate seven core practices that enable Labor-Management Partnerships to achieve and sustain highly positive outcomes. We have provided information to demonstrate how these practices have been implemented in the two settings, information that we will address in more detail in the following chapter.

Although these central practices might be difficult to implement in all Labor-Management Partnerships, it is important to understand how each helps to shape and then sustain a successful process (see figure 3). Once the rationale for each practice is understood, organizations can creatively explore how to fit them into their particular culture, bud get, and need.

Lastly, it is important to develop a succession planning process to smoothly transfer responsibilities to newly appointed management and union leaders as the Partnership process matures. It takes time to significantly alter the culture of an organization to fully support worker participation initiatives. Continuing to nurture such a culture is extremely important, requiring ongoing education of new entries into the system about the values and practices of such a culture. Particularly when senior managers at the union and administrative levels change, it is crucial to carefully introduce them into the ongoing Partnership process. The challenge facing healthcare organizations is to make performance gains "permanent" by hardwiring the learning from individual projects and initiatives into the way the organization does business. Continued progress will also require deepening levels of teamwork, developing more data systems, and evaluating progress to ensure that changes really are producing the intended results.[129]

Figure 3. Starting a Labor-Management Transformation Process

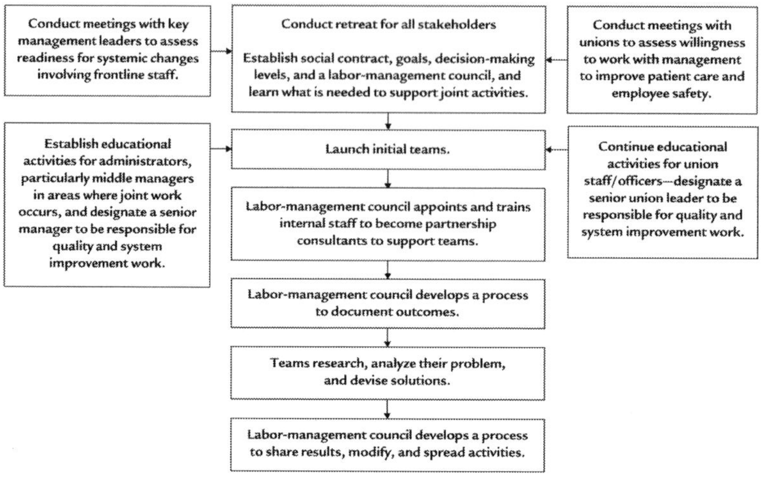

CHAPTER 4

Team Structures for Frontline Staff Participation

> Effectively, change is almost impossible without ... collaboration, cooperation and consensus.
>
> —*Simon Mainwaring*

In chapter 1, we described the evolution of worker participation activities in the United States. The three basic structures used in this pursuit have been unit-based teams, departmental teams, and intensive Study Action Teams, more recently established within structured Labor-Management Partnership (LMP) processes.

Since many union and management leaders are not aware of their choices in structuring and deepening their Partnership process, this chapter provides further details about the inner workings of the three different approaches.[130] Making an informed choice about the structure of joint work is particularly important for organizations with limited staff time, so that they can make the best use of their resources.

In presenting the options of different structures, we stress that it is a challenge for healthcare institutions, or for most organizations for that matter, to jump immediately into a complex and broad engagement process such as departmental and intensive Study Action Teams without adequate preparation.[131] Luckily, employee participation processes can be approached with an initial series of shallow dives, rather than beginning with a leap from the high-diving board. Some organizations may find it most cost-effective to choose these less complicated options for their purposes.

Unit-Based Teams

Unit-based teams enable labor and management to focus on issues they agree upon as representing discrete, solvable patient care problems. As such, they represent an excellent means of initiating a worker participation process. They provide frontline staff with a direct role in improving both care and working conditions in a particular work area.

Many partnerships function successfully at a contained, unit-based level. At Kaiser, unit-based teams have remained the predominant and preferred method of frontline staff participation, obtaining significant improvements in patient care, patient safety, and staff safety, and in achieving more meaningful jobs.[132]

An example of a successful unit-based team is the Laboratory team at Maimonides Medical Center, one of the first projects of their Partnership process. This unit-based team was composed of lab technicians and their supervisor working in the laboratory that analyzed both inpatient and outpatient blood samples. Marie-Cecile Charlier, a lab technician and a key member of this team, viewed unit-based teams as important vehicles for improving the flexibility and effectiveness of the lab and for improving staff morale. For years, Charlier had suggested to upper management ways to achieve better efficiency in lab operations, but her suggestions were routinely ignored. "Finally, we had a chance to be heard,"[133] commented Charlier when asked why she decided to join the laboratory's unit-based team. When she learned about the new Partnership activities planned at Maimonides, Charlier became guardedly optimistic that she and other co-workers might finally find a real voice for decision making, or at least for offering input, about their unit.

Once the Maimonides Strategic Alliance Council identified the lab as one of the first unit-based areas for work, Charlier encouraged six other lab technicians to work with her to evaluate and propose improvements for the lab's operations. She was able to do this fairly easily, since Charlier, a natural leader, was known for her energy, for her respect for her co-workers, and for her integrity. Absolutely serious about and committed to her job, Charlier also spent her spare time working with community arts and cultural organizations. When she suggested that they join, her co-workers did so readily. Her lab supervisor, on the other hand, agreed to join the team somewhat reluctantly. She made it clear that she didn't feel the staff could contribute any practical insights for improving lab effectiveness but eventually agreed to participate in this "experiment."[134]

To help this unit-based team get started, a member of the Labor-Management Project from SEIU 1199[135] provided problem-solving and conflict-resolution strategies and tools to analyze the departmental workflow and the layout of their equipment. Lazes encouraged the team to create ground rules for working together that could serve to minimize any disruptive or distracting behavior within the team.

The team's initial goal was broadly framed: "To increase staff flexibility and reduce turnaround time." While reducing turnaround time was a goal that might be planned for and measured, "increasing staff flexibility" was quite vague. Realizing this, the team spent the first two meetings assessing what might represent a solvable approach to obviously low staff morale. They identified a particularly loaded issue: virtually all staff members were upset at having to work at least one weekend per month and several holidays each year. The team became convinced that this scheduling problem could be resolved and that doing so would improve staff morale and productivity.

One of the team's first activities involved collecting data on current turnaround time for getting lab results back to clinicians in the Emergency Department (ED). The ED turnaround time was not consistent: the average return was measured at 1 hour but could reach 1½ to 2 hours. Reducing laboratory turnaround was important for ED patients, particularly those patients in critical condition. After consulting with lab staff from all shifts, the team concluded that it was realistic to try to reduce this time to under 30 minutes. To accomplish this, team members solicited suggestions for changes from lab and ED staff. At the same time, two team members were assigned to research articles about methods used in other settings to reduce laboratory test turnaround time. The entire team then carefully reviewed all of this data.

After the initial team meetings, Marie-Cecile Charlier was elected as the team leader. Her responsibilities involved creating the agenda for each meeting in consultation with the other team members, keeping basic notes of decisions made at each meeting, making sure that follow-up assignments were completed, and checking with all team members and invited guests to ensure that they could attend the weekly meetings. After analyzing the research articles and data collected from lab staff about the current process, the team was prepared to contemplate potential changes.

Before finalizing their recommendations, however, they requested the opportunity to test new equipment they had learned about and to perform a modest redesign of their lab based on their workflow analysis. Having conducted multiple tests of each, after three months of work the team offered its recommendations. These included redesigning the layout of lab equipment to maximize the use of each workstation; purchasing new equipment that was easier to use and required fewer reagents; cross-training the staff so that they could perform all lab tests rather than just the ones they had previously been assigned, thus increasing efficiency and expanding job descriptions; increasing compensation so that each lab staff member would be paid for becoming multiskilled; moving phlebotomists from the laboratory to the ED so that blood could be drawn more quickly; and hiring additional part-time staff so that full-time staff wouldn't need to work weekends and holidays.

When the lab team presented their recommendations to senior managers and labor leaders, all were accepted, and a sidebar agreement was created to guarantee that employees would have opportunities for training to perform multiple tests and receive compensation for these new responsibilities. It took the hospital a little over two months to renovate the laboratory and another month to accomplish cross-training, recruit new parttime staff, and obtain new equipment.

As a result of this unit-based team's work, turnaround times for test results transmitted to the ER were reduced to less than 30 minutes. In fact, similar turnaround times were achieved for all hospital departments once phlebotomists were assigned directly to each hospital department. Staff morale soared as a result of these improvements and of eliminating weekend and holiday shifts.

After working on the lab team and seeing its impact, Charlier became eager to spread worker participation opportunities at Maimonides. Pam Brier and John Reid soon recruited her for the new role of Developer (internal consultant) for the hospital. They had witnessed Charlier in action: she was clearly an employee with considerable skills and a passion for partnership activities and for improving patient care. Several years later, Charlier was elected as a vice president of SEIU 1199 representing workers at Maimonides. Each of these positions enabled her to continue encouraging and supporting worker participation activities.

Department-Based Study Groups

In 2005, six unexpected fatalities occurred in the Maimonides Cardiology Department's four inpatient units. An initial investigation by hospital administrators and risk management staff (the group assigned to investigate troubling clinical outcomes) concluded that each incident occurred after a significant delay in response to cardiac telemetry monitor alarms. Two nurses were blamed for causing several of the deaths through lateness in responding to these alarms and were suspended until the investigation was completed.

When Veronica Richardson, shop steward for the nurses (New York State Nurses Association), and

Marie-Cecile Charlier, now a Developer and an SEIU 1199 shop steward,[136] learned of the suspensions, they and other colleagues requested that the executive director of the Cardiology Department, Louise Valero, initiate a process to identify the root causes of the fatal delays. This would require a department-wide, systemic approach rather than a unit-based study. Shifting from unit-based work to departmental LMP teams was already being contemplated at Maimonides, but the seriousness of the situation in Cardiology hastened this decision for both the administration and the Cardiology staff.

The Cardiology Department Labor-Management Committee was formed in 2006 to analyze all facets of the issues that led to the six deaths. In addition to Marie-Cecile Charlier and Veronica Richardson, 12 other members composed the department-based work group. These included Cardiology interns and residents, nurse practitioners, physician assistants, attending physicians, nurses, patient care technicians, ward clerks, and transporters for cardiac patients. Team members included employees from all four cardiac units (Intensive Care and three "step-down" units). Evening and night-shift staff members attended the weekly group meetings, receiving overtime pay for coming in early or staying late in order to participate.

The first tasks for the committee included a literature review of methods utilized elsewhere for reducing time to respond to cardiac monitors, a review of the data from the Risk Management Department of the circumstances surrounding the recent fatalities, and the tracking of response times to alarms and monitors in all cardiac units for one month. Staff on all shifts were interviewed to identify any difficulties they had with the current cardiac alarm systems.

Two major issues became apparent from the data collected and from staff interviews: the nursing staff had difficulty in accurately setting patients' cardiac alarms, and they lacked a standard process for determining acuity levels across all cardiac units. (An acuity level determines the extent of nursing assistance that a patient requires, which in turn affects the number of patients assigned to any nurse, and thus their workload.) Other problems that were identified were difficulty in hearing alarms from the cardiac monitors at the nurses' stations, and lack of staff qualified to respond to monitors or to assess patients' cardiac status as they transported patients to tests outside their immediate units.

While this departmental team met biweekly to discuss the details of the ongoing analysis, a smaller work group compiled findings from their research and interviews to pre sent to the larger group. This work group included Agnes Aban, a dedicated nurse, shy but determined, who found strength in representing her unit in this department-wide team; Maureen O'Neil, a nurse practitioner, a natural, respected leader whose lovely sense of humor paired with great discipline; and Ron Barranco, a thoughtful nurse who helped encourage employees who were too shy to speak up.

Veronica Richardson and Marie-Cecile Charlier, with Louise Valero, RN, the charismatic and strong-willed executive director of Cardiac Services, provided support for the overall project and attended most of the smaller work group meetings. The director of Organizational Performance and the director of Risk Management also worked with the team and eventually helped track outcomes of their recommendations as they were implemented.

Reaching a consensus on standardizing acuity levels for all four units was a particular challenge for this team, due to its size and the diversity of its staff. Some physicians and physician assistants on the team were initially reluctant to engage in such a process. Each practitioner felt it important to "have the freedom as professionals" to determine how much nursing care was needed for their patient. "This is what we are trained to do: to make clinical judgments," contended one clinician in discussing the controversy.

After several meetings of the entire committee during which this matter was debated, Charlier and Valero decided to meet with these practitioners individually. They discussed the rationale for standardizing acuity levels and the importance of this work for the nursing staff. Charlier and Valero carefully listened to each of the staff members' concerns and eventually crafted and presented a proposal to the team that incorporated feedback from these meetings.

The process of being heard and of having their suggestions incorporated into the final proposal led these clinicians to endorse and support the final agreement. Three acuity levels would be established for each of the four cardiac units. Each physician, resident, or physician assistant responsible for a particular patient would evaluate general risk factors and individualized considerations in order to determine one of the three levels for that patient. Nurses' assignments—and thus their daily workload—would then be determined by the acuity levels of the patients on each unit.

After meeting for three months and consulting with other co-workers, the departmental team recommended five changes: (1) purchasing new telemetry equipment that nurses could more easily adjust; (2) holding interdisciplinary rounds at the start of each shift to clarify or adjust patient acuity levels and to recheck the alarm settings on all telemetry equipment; (3) reducing noise at the nurses' stations by forbidding unnecessary conversations in these areas so that patient call bells and telemetry alarms could be better heard; (4) requiring a licensed independent practitioner (LIP) to accompany an acuity level 3 patient (the most critical patients) being transferred in or out of the units; and (5) conducting in-service training for nurses on properly setting and performing minor repairs to the telemetry monitors, as well as recognizing which readings required immediate responses from unit physicians.

It took several months to implement all five recommendations. To follow up the project's results, the hospital's Department of Organizational Performance designed an effective tool, which the team accepted, for collecting future data on alarm response times on all four units.

Overall response time to cardiac monitor alarms has stayed consistently at or below 1 minute since this project's recommendations were implemented, as opposed to between 2.5 and 8 minutes previously. Notably, there have been no adverse patient events due to delayed alarm responses on these units since the project was completed in 2007.[137]

"The interdisciplinary team approach to extremely serious problems in the Cardiology Department far exceeded our expectations. The Departmental Labor Management Committee strengthened relationships among all care providers, in addition to its other impressive results. The project will serve as the model for future departmental collaboration and for all subsequent joint work with the departments of Organizational Performance and Risk Management,"[138] Louise Valero emphasized when interviewed a few months after the implementation of the team's recommendations. This departmental team continues to initiate other projects within Cardiology, addressing other patient care issues.

While a unit-based team structure focuses on the concerns of individual units, departmental Partnership structures strengthen inter-unit functionality within a department and between departments. This approach also helped the Medical Center to maximize limited resources.[139] "It was an important decision to refocus our Partnership activities from discrete unit-based projects to departmental activities. We had limited resources and wanted to make sure we used them most effectively. We also saw that many of the problems identified within our units overlapped with others within their department. So, we wanted to be sure we had the most effective structures in place to help get at the bottom of all these issues,"[140] explained Pam Brier, former CEO and president of Maimonides.

As a result of the impressive outcomes of the Cardiology Alarm/Monitor project, the federal Medicare oversight group MedPAC requested a presentation on this approach, which was made in October 2008 in Washington, DC.[141]

Study Action Teams

As stated in chapter 1, the intensive Study Action Team (SAT) is employed to create breakthroughs that result in new systemwide structures and processes. This approach is now a proven strategy for companies and healthcare organizations to use when they recognize that significant changes are needed, but the end goal is not yet clear.[142]

Initially implemented at Xerox with their union ACTWU, a Study Action Team process enabled the company to achieve plant-wide changes[143] during a critical time.[144] As noted in chapter 1, the Xerox SAT process saved the company $3.7 million and avoided a layoff of 180 employees. The process resulted in an overall 28 percent reduction in manufacturing costs.[145] To fully understand how the Study Action Team process worked, some background information about Xerox's Labor-Management Partnership will provide a context.

Xerox had initiated a robust Labor-Management Partnership in 1980, and by 1981 over 19 percent of their workforce was engaged in some form of worker participation activity.[146] At the end of 1981, a new challenge arose. A year-long secret study by a strategic planning team of engineers and financial analysts revealed that several Xerox copiers were no longer competitive because of the high cost of some of their component parts. In the preceding years, competition had intensified with companies like Ricoh, Sharp, and Canon in Japan and with Kodak and IBM in the United States. Xerox's market share had dropped from 90 percent to 43 percent by the early 1980s.[147] The confidential report suggested that to remain competitive in the United States, Xerox needed to start manufacturing component copier parts in Mexico, where labor costs were significantly lower.

These parts would then be transported to the United States for assembly, so that Xerox copiers could still be advertised as "manufactured in the U.S." The first copier component selected for manufacture in Mexico was the wire harness. This is the section of Xerox copiers in which all the internal wires come together through an expensive and complex manufacturing process.

As the labor-management consultant working with Xerox and the ACTWU union at the time, Lazes discovered this internal report from informal conversations with several engineers while exploring ways for them to work with the current problem-solving teams. He was given a copy, and immediately after reading it, requested meetings with key union and management leaders: Tony Costanza (general shop chairman of AC-TWU), Les Calder (vice president for the Xerox division of ACTWU), Bill Asher (vice president for labor relations for Xerox), and David Kearns (CEO and president of Xerox). After individual discussions with each leader, he organized a joint meeting with all four. In a private meeting with Asher, he had stressed that it might be unwise for the union to try to solve the huge cost-reduction goal, as he thought it unlikely to be achievable without significant wage and benefit reductions. Asher felt that engaging the union in a "doomed" process might jeopardize Xerox's good relationship with ACTWU and reduce the union's willingness to participate further in joint activities. The union leaders, on the other hand, felt that the workers deserved to try to discover ways to reduce production costs and, by doing so, to save the 180 jobs.

While these discussions were taking place, Lazes spent time conversing with production workers and engineers about methods to achieve extensive cost savings. Cross-departmental work groups alone seemed unlikely to achieve the necessary results. He felt out on a limb, since he now had persuaded both labor and management to work jointly on finding ways to avoid this layoff: What kind of process should be employed? While jogging one morning before reporting to the Xerox plant, he flashed on a potential solution: to create a special team of frontline workers, managers, and technical advisers who would be reassigned to work full-time for six months on an extensive cost-saving analysis.

The engineers with whom he discussed this plan thought it was a long shot, as they had already spent a year themselves trying to find a solution. Nonetheless, they felt that the new Study Action Team idea might enable more outside-the-box thinking. The new work group not only would have the opportunity to redesign the production process but also could suggest changes in equipment, supplies, and actual job structures. Further, it could suggest changes to the company's contract with the union, something that had been off-limits to the engineers during their initial analysis. The engineers acknowledged, too, that the frontline production workers actually knew more than they did about which practical changes might be feasible. Their guarded yet positive feedback gave me the confidence to suggest the new, more far-reaching participation process to Asher, Calder, Costanza, and Kearns.

After several meetings, Lazes persuaded them to establish this innovative strategy. The process would enable frontline staff and the union to have a direct role in finding ways to save their jobs, rather than to simply react defensively to a management proposal. Although senior management remained concerned that the new process might jeopardize their relationship with the union, the workforce agreed to go forward with the new team process. It was stated clearly that if this work group couldn't achieve the needed cost savings, management would need to implement a layoff.

Management and union leaders decided upon a full-time team of six production workers, one engineer, and the supervisor for the wire harness area to compose the new work group. More than 160 production workers from the Components Manufacturing Operations (CMO) plant applied to become members. Calder and Costanza, along with several shop stewards, interviewed all of the candidates for this project. Job criteria included having participated on a current problem-solving team, demonstrating excellent communication and writing skills, possessing knowledge of the current contract, showing evidence of strategic or analytical thinking, and being well-respected by their peers.

The team's task was defined by a new sidebar agreement to the existing contract: it would seek "to find ways to be competitive, improve quality, cost and delivery performance of the business to levels which will assure a positive competitive position and ultimately, to secure jobs."[148] It was understood that if their eventual proposal involved new job responsibilities or other changes that affected the collective bargaining agreement with the union, management and union leaders would need to agree to these changes before their implementation.

During the initial week of the SAT process, the team spent time strengthening problem-solving and communications skills, discussing how best to work together and how to divide up their tasks. They developed a strategy of actively engaging all plant employees, soliciting their suggestions and encouraging their support. Work group members met with the plant's finance staff to establish a focus on areas in the production process that could yield the greatest cost reductions. The finance staff also provided information about Xerox's accounting process and the basic financial methods used to calculate production costs.

An Executive Labor-Management Oversight Committee was formed to assist the Study Action Team process, composed of local and national union leaders and Xerox executives. This group provided technical assistance to the team and ensured that they would have access to critical data about production costs and to any staff whom they desired to meet: production workers, engineers, managers, equipment vendors, and others. The Oversight Committee was given the ultimate authority on contractual language changes and for securing funds to purchase new equipment. The need for this executive committee was anticipated from the start, as it was likely that the Study Action Team's recommendations would need approval beyond the authority of local management and labor leaders at the CMO manufacturing plant.

From the beginning, the Study Action Team members actively solicited ideas and information from all employees about their work responsibilities, workflow through the plant, the quality of supplier parts, and the efficiency of current equipment. Over their six months of work, the SAT kept frontline staff, engineers, and managers of the CMO plant informed of their progress and continued soliciting their feedback, knowing that this process of connecting to frontline staff would be crucial for the eventual acceptance of any recommendations.

Key areas for improvement that the team explored included potential purchasing and layout of new equipment, changes in the assembly processes, new sources for component parts for assembling the wire harness, and a more effective use of space in the CMO. The team made weekly "walk-around visits" to the wire harness production department to apprise the production workers there of their ongoing analysis and to ask questions. However, since they were contemplating significant changes in the overall manufacturing process, in the purchase of new equipment, and in the responsibilities of hourly employees and management, the team agreed that until there was agreement on their final proposal, their final recommendations would remain confidential. This was important because every aspect of the final proposal would depend on the acceptance of the other proposed changes, so discussing a particular component of a potential solution in isolation would be counterproductive.

In addition to extensive engagement with all wire harness department workers, members of the Study Action Team visited competitors to learn how they organized the manufacturing of similar parts. Several of these trips were made to nonunion plants that used very different production methods and equipment. In considering new equipment, the study team had production workers test the equipment on a trial basis to evaluate whether it reduced costs and increased efficiency.

After six months of analysis and proposal development, the SAT provided data to support 40 recommendations for producing a higher quality, more cost-efficient wire harness. The key categories of recommendations included (1) purchasing new equipment to assemble the wire harness faster and more efficiently; (2) changing suppliers to ensure a higher quality of component parts—this would reduce the need for rework and thus achieve significant cost savings; (3)

rearranging equipment and parts bins so that employees could reduce wasted time accessing parts while assembling the wire harness; and (4) creating self-managing work groups instead of the existing production line process, reducing the need for rework and making employees' jobs more interesting. Adopting this new work structure meant that employees could easily switch jobs as needed whenever changes in production schedules or in product mixes dictated this. Lastly (5), overhead costs were reduced by consolidating the assembly process in one section of the CMO building. The SAT identified total cost savings amounting to $3.7 million, or $500,000 more than the agreed-upon target.[149]

After several work sessions with the Executive Labor-Management Oversight Committee to review and analyze the recommendations, senior labor and management leaders accepted all recommendations and agreed to make specific changes to the collective bargaining agreement that would enable frontline staff to work in the new production work groups and to receive compensation for becoming multiskilled.

It took several months to fully implement the SAT recommendations. "When fully in place, this process succeeded far beyond everyone's expectations and opened up major possibilities for new ways of having labor and management work together. We realized that this process could continue helping us to improve the quality of parts and to reduce costs in our manufacturing division,"[150] commented Bill Asher,

Xerox's vice president for labor relations and an important SAT adviser. As result of the team's success, Xerox decided to use a similar process to evaluate all other component parts assembly methods for their copiers.[151]

The impressive results of the Xerox Study Action Teams were described in journal articles, books, and newspapers, including a special report by the U.S. Department of Labor.[152] Several U.S. manufacturing companies began to employ Study Action Teams to reduce costs, improve product quality, and save the jobs of American workers.[153]

Although the SAT process was initially established in manufacturing companies to obtain cost and quality outcomes, this method has now been used to improve patient satisfaction, cost-effectiveness, and quality of care in healthcare systems.[154]

Summary

Choosing among the different structures of Labor-Management Partnerships described previously should be guided by the characteristics and situations of each organization: shaped by its particular needs and values, by the attitudes of its union partner(s), by its management culture, and by the existing relationship between the two. In some organizations, an entrenched, adversarial relationship between labor and management makes partnerships difficult if not impossible. When labor and management are willing to invest in finding ways to work together, however, such activities can achieve impressive results (see table 3).[155]

Implementing Labor-Management Partnership initiatives in healthcare and in other organizations is an evolving process. Beginning with one approach doesn't preclude shifting to another over time to adjust to new needs.

Kaiser Permanente, Maimonides Medical Center, Hathaway shirt company, and Xerox Corporation Partnerships all demonstrated a flexible approach to their Partnership work as their process matured and as they continued to respond to the changing needs of their patients or customers.

Table3. Comparing Forms of Worker Participation Activities

Forms of Involvement	Best Use/Benefits	Resources Needed	Level of Difficulty	Estimated Time for Staff	Examples
Unit-based	Unit-based quality and process improvement activities	Basic support	Low	Two hours/week	Allegheny General Hospital, Los Angeles Department of Health Services, Kaiser Maimonides, and Kaiser

Forms of Involvement	Best Use/Benefits	Resources Needed	Level of Difficulty	Estimated Time for Staff	Examples
Departmental	Improving interfaces between groups within a department	Basic support	Low	Two hours/month	Maimonides
Study Action Teams	Creating new work systems	Significant support	High	Full time for three to four months	Maimonides and Xerox

As stated earlier in this chapter, many of the initial Labor-Management Partnerships focused on shop floor and then departmental problem-solving teams, yet there is increasing awareness that for future Labor-Management Partnerships to be effective, particularly in healthcare organizations where many see disruptive innovation as necessary,[156] they need to focus on both *shop floor and strategic/systemic* activities. Regardless of the approach used, we need to continue working on ways to improve how care is delivered.

Also, whether in restructuring the manufacturing process at the Hathaway shirt company or shifting to an integrated healthcare delivery system in the Los Angeles County Department of Health Services, unions have played a strategic role in organizational decision making, helping to make these organizations more effective and efficient. The involvement of national unions has enabled several Labor-Management Partnerships to secure financial and at times technical resources to help sustain and spread Labor-Management Partnerships. At LA-DHS, SEIU 721 helped to expand the ability of L.A. County to obtain Medicaid funds to pay for uninsured patients and funds for staff retraining.

Establishing a high-involvement work system is much easier when a new organization is created: in organizations like Saturn and at some Volvo plants. These organizations generally have fewer of the constraints inherent in an existing culture or long-favored but no longer efficient work practices. Shifting or transforming existing organizations to more effective ones is clearly more complicated than starting from scratch; unfortunately, most of us don't have the opportunity to start from scratch. In these situations, collaborative leadership interventions—combined with a felt necessity—can help create openness to new ways of working. A collaborative leadership process can lend legitimacy to a new partnership. However, labor and management leaders need to keep in mind that in both new and traditional organizations, it is essential not to get too far ahead, too quickly, of what either frontline staff or management can accept, or resistance to change will occur. The particular challenges associated with creating a Labor-Management Partnership process within an existing organization are presented in chapter 8.

CHAPTER 5

Challenges in Labor-Management Work Groups

> Groups ... set imperceptible limits to their thinking, while sabotaging ideas that do not conform.
>
> —*Ken Eisold*

Thus far we have provided a socio-technical systems (STS) model for organizational change. As we described earlier, this model grew out of a psychodynamic group relations approach pioneered by Wilfred Bion and refined and practiced since at the Tavistock Institute in London. Eric Trist and Fred Emery adapted that model, incorporating emerging insights from operations research, systems theory, and participative management practices and from the writing of Kurt Lewin, an American social scientist and field theorist. Fred Emery and Einar Thorsrud further developed the approach, which spread rapidly across Western Europe and Scandinavia, and into Australia. The STS model emphasizes facilitating communication within and among multiple levels in hierarchical systems. It aims to merge the social and technical dimensions of work life, and to foster democracy in the workplace.[157]

We have been convinced of the utility of both the sociotechnical and group psychodynamic perspectives, which we see as complementary.[158] The psychodynamic group relations model that evolved at Tavistock offers insight into subjective experiences of group members as they encounter the social forces specific to group life. Knowledge of these forces is useful in mentoring group leaders, internal consultants, and team members about the undercurrents in group mood that can distract members from working on their common task.

Consultants from both socio-technical and group psychoanalytic backgrounds[159] tend to agree on the processes and structures that benefit group cohesion and task performance. These include the selection, at least initially, of motivated, socially adept members; training these members in problem-solving and conflict-resolution skills; and adopting a clear working methodology. Consultants from each perspective emphasize that effective leadership, the encouragement of task participation by all group members, and the establishment of clear and achievable goals help working groups to remain task focused. With these safeguards, groups become more than the sum of their parts, with the potential for great creativity.

Without a clear working structure, on the other hand, groups tend to implode into infighting or attacking "outsiders" as a way to maintain their own unity, or into rigid stances that are not based on a realistic appraisal of their circumstances. Group psychodynamic theory and practice offer a window into why groups can be vulnerable to such *regressions:* that is, why groups are prone at times to retreat into unproductive mindsets, emotionally fraught interactions, or highly unrealistic choices. Kenneth Eisold,[160] an experienced group-analytic consultant, notes that upon entering a group, members at the outset will tend to appraise and lump people into categories (e.g., "She is like me," "He is not like me," "She is boring," "He is a pushover," "She is the popular one," "He is too aggressive"). They continue to make such appraisals in order to grasp the shifting complexities of the group as it evolves, to find a way to secure a position in the group hierarchy. Individuals sense that others are categorizing them, too, and fear being misunderstood, stereo typed, or left without allies.

The social pressures of finding a way to belong, to be understood and effective within the group, can push members to become judgmental and overly competitive, or passive, guarded, and watchful, depending on their temperaments, personalities, and personal histories. Because of these forces at play within their membership, groups can swing into disruptive emotional states until they begin to trust their leader, the other group members, and their work itself. When groups do become captured by one dominant emotion or another (such as rage, euphoria, or suspiciousness), their members become increasingly insecure, struggle to understand what is happening, and can feel pressed into taking on roles that confuse them, such as participating in bullying.[161]

"Regressive" Group Functioning

One of the first practitioners to study and identify such confusing and unproductive forces in groups was Wilfred Bion, a British psychiatrist who led and studied groups of soldiers hospitalized with "battle fatigue" during World War II. Bion discovered that when he maintained silence in order to encourage the soldiers' contributions to group therapy sessions, the group members, experiencing themselves as "leaderless," reverted to one of three characteristic positions. They began to fight with their leader, with an internal subgroup seen as "to blame" for the group's difficulties in working on their problems, or with "outsiders" whom they blamed for their own struggles or whose power they feared. (Bion termed these "fight-flight" groups.)

Alternatively, a group could become passively dependent, failing to make their own creative contributions to the joint discussions and essentially leaving the group's work solely to their leader. Such groups tend to be either hostile toward their task and their leader or overidealize his or her capacities. Bion called this phenomenon "dependency group" functioning.

Finally, groups might alleviate their discomfort by engaging in gossipy, distracting conversations about famous personalities, often with sexual innuendos, or even speculate about romantic attachments or alliances within pairs in their group.

Bion intuited that the common theme behind such conversations was the hope that by thus distracting themselves, the group members might magically escape the burden of their work, of internal group conflicts, or of the pressure to belong. (He called these "pairing groups.") Some group members utilize such gossipy interchanges to connect, or pair, with other members.

The term "regressions," used by Bion for such dominant group moods and modes of functioning, is a psychoanalytic one. It refers to the fact that people, when faced with difficulties that remind them even obliquely of previous times when they felt helpless, full of conflict, and alone, may begin to behave in a manner that is not tied to their current reality. Instead, they "regress" to thoughts and feelings that are determined more by those prior difficulties than by their pre sent situation. For example, they may feel more angry or depressed or frozen than their current experience seems to merit. Bion observed that similar regressions occur in groups, too, stimulated by the difficulties inherent in group membership but also by matters such as the particular *context* of the group (that is, the group's role and relationship within a larger organization), by their particular *task* (e.g., how difficult or controversial it might be), and by their group's *history.*

To Bion's descriptions of these common regressive modes of functioning, social scientist Earl Hopper[162] added another type—"massification," or the group's adoption of a rigid "party line," expressed largely in jargon or cliché. Such groups tend to extrude members immediately when they do not adhere to the party line, which only aggravates a sense of danger, both external and internal to the group.

Roger Shapiro, commenting on the tendency for groups to regress, noted that these tendencies to compete, to fight, to flee, or to search for a sense of connection can actually be motivating factors in group life as long as they do not completely distract the group from their task.[163] For Shapiro, a skillful leader can sense the direction of the group's energies and can influence them or in turn be influenced by the group's mood to change course.

Strengthening Leadership: Speaking to the Mood of the Group

Effective leaders often intuitively sense the mood of their group and articulate or in some way respond to their under lying fears or wishes. *The constructive use of a group's regressive energies can powerfully motivate members toward a cooperative, enthusiastic tackling of their task.* For example, a leader responding to her group's functioning in a "dependency" mode might speak empathically to a group's desires for the "answers" they expect "higher-ups" to provide them while saying something like, "I get it. Management is being paid to come up with solutions to this; we are not." The leader might at the same time remind the group, however, "The administration knows about costs and regulations, but *we* know about actual clinical practice. We can come up with solutions they don't really have the experience to figure out. It will make our lives easier, and the patients will get better care if we can do this." In this way, the leader may gently shift the group from a dependent to a more competitive stance.

Further examples of *responding to a group's mood to promote a task-focus* include:[164]

1. Employing a stance of active listening to every member's input can allay group members' fears of being unheard or steamrolled by the group or by its leader. In chapter 4, we provided an example of this when we described the decision made by Maimonides Cardiology team leaders to meet privately with physicians and physician assistants on their team in order to better understand and address their concerns, while also explaining the importance of the group's meeting the strongly expressed needs of the nursing staff.

2. In addition to active listening, the leader also needs to defuse any emerging discontent about her capacity to reconcile opposing viewpoints once they are voiced and heard. The action mentioned previously by the Cardiology team leaders led to a workable compromise that satisfied all factions of their work group and enabled the team to move forward.

3. Demonstrating a grounded sense of excitement, expectation and a realistic hopefulness about the group's work may counter unrealistic flights of group fancy, while still encouraging their optimism. A leader might thus say, "Hey, I think we are onto something here! But how can we take this idea and make it actually work in practice?"

4. The leader's attitude can also help to counter any tendency toward clichéd groupthink. When a leader recognizes that her group is starting to speak in jargon and has stopped thinking creatively about potential solutions, she may interject a question such as, "I'm not sure that we are getting to the bottom of things here. I think we need to unpack these assumptions a bit more."

The Consultant’s Role in Assisting Team Leaders

Working with a team that is enthusiastic, well-structured, and motivated is delightful: in these instances, the group becomes truly more than the sum of its parts and the joint work becomes deeply satisfying and exciting. However, groups may also become stuck in one or another regressive mood and mode of functioning, and this may be disorienting to the group leader, who can become unsure about how to proceed. When consulting to the designated leader of such a team, the consultant should first ask the leader to examine whether or not the group has a clear understanding of its task, senses that it can be accomplished within the time provided, and thinks that it is worthwhile. Without this basic grounding, most groups will become stuck and reactive. The work group leader should be encouraged to confer with her team to clarify their understanding of team goals, of whether or not they feel they are relevant and achievable, and of their overall direction. If it emerges that the group concerns are based on factors such as a lack of adequate time or resources, the team leader should speak with a representative of the committee directing Partnership activities about this situation.

If there is an under lying controversy among team members about the group’s purpose or methods, this needs to be addressed directly by the leader with all team members. Burying a disagreement about a central task issue will backfire, as a subgroup of members will inevitably feel unheard and lose trust in their leader's and group members' ability to withstand conflict.[165]

If members' concerns about their goals seem to result from a misunderstanding of the task itself or from a kind of regression described previously, the leader needs to enlist the alliance of group members who seem to understand the task and to be evaluating it realistically, to draw them out about their thinking. After allowing discussion, the leader, in conjunction with these team members, should propose a potential solution or assign one of these members to seek out factual material about the controversy before the next meeting.

Consultants should sit in on group meetings from time to time to gauge their under lying mood. Specifically: Is the team passively acquiescent? Engaged in in-group or intra-group fighting? Spinning its wheels with gossip or with overly optimistic ideas that seem unlikely to gain traction? The consultant can then help the group leader to identify the under lying mood and to find ways of redirecting it, as described previously.

If the internal consultant finds that the group is working on either a task that lacks importance or on a solution that seems likely to be in effective, it is important that he or she discuss this with the group leader. In a study[166] in which Rudden examined videotapes of work groups at Maimonides, it became obvious that most unit-based groups chose a central problem in clinical care delivery to research and to solve. One group, however, selected an issue that was secondary to other pressing clinical concerns and then approached their study in a superficial manner. This occurred toward the beginning of the Labor-Management Partnership and may have reflected a misunderstanding of the process on the part of this group leader, leaving her team to produce a poster presentation rather than a substantive solution to a clinical issue. Such a choice may have also represented a "protective" measure to avoid encountering a central, but more divisive, clinical care issue. An experienced consultant would want to describe to such a work group leader the kinds of projects other groups were undertaking and to help her to encourage the group to work on a problem with greater potential.

The consultant should also try to discern whether the leader is out of step with, or unaware of, the culture of the group membership. Some academics studying leadership have focused on the match between the group's and leader's motivations and culture.[167] Without understanding divisive forces already at play in a group (often related to hierarchy, differences in member cultures and ethnicities, or prior experiences in the overall organization), the leader will not be prepared to surmount these preexisting difficulties. Further, because group fears and concerns can limit what the group can achieve, both leader and consultant need to gauge the group's readiness to perform their task.[168]

It is important that the work group leader recognize any difficulties imposed by meeting times or by the additional demands of group work over and above members' scheduled work hours. It is also vital to directly address members' reservations about cooperating with management or staff. Usually, preliminary training in conflict resolution and problem solving can help prepare group members for the job, but sometimes the leader must work on understanding negative attitudes in the group about their joint work. Historical frictions among representatives of different units, disciplines, or ethnic groups may need to be recognized and addressed. How to work with such frictions will be delineated via an example later in this chapter.

The consultant should further mentor leaders whose group's work has stalled due to an actively dissenting team subgroup. Such subgroups tend to be led by one or two individuals who strongly express a particular disagreement about the workings of the team. Bion observed that the nominal leader of a group is not always the de facto leader. Roger Shapiro, mentioned earlier, underscored this idea by emphasizing that the group leader can only *actually* lead after having gained the support of at least some members of the dissenting subgroup.[169] If he or she cannot, then the person who best captures the dominant group mood may seize implicit or explicit control of the team.

A leadership coach or consultant needs to approach such a situation carefully, realizing that *a fractious subgroup is usually expressing a part of the group's experience that needs to be understood and acknowledged.* Effective leaders search for what is important in a subgroup's message, actively listen to it, and address it before trying to redirect the group's energies. This is crucial to the group's ability to regain its task focus.

A somewhat different situation occurs when the dissenting subgroup is led by an individual member who herself experiences difficulty with groups and seems to repeatedly place herself at the center of controversy. Such an individual may be convinced that she will never be recognized or allowed to make an impact without aggressive self-assertion. Alternatively, the member may be intensely competitive or convinced, in a grandiose way, that she is "the only one with the answers." At times, such a member may be unable to absorb other people's points of view, to think about and learn from them, because of her urgent need for visibility and praise.

If a member is continually disruptive, leading a number of dissenting subgroups, one after another, then the group leader should meet with him or her individually to describe the problem, acknowledging the validity of some points the member raises, but *reiterating the values of the group about collaboration and mutual learning.* In a Partnership, a fellow labor representative should preferably attend this conversation. If this intervention does not improve the situation, the work group member should be told that his or her input into organizational change would be better expressed in a different venue and be helped to find an alternative situation that is a better fit.

Cultivating Alternate Leaders

Labor-Management Partnerships that practice collaborative leadership are structured to explicitly value each employee's knowledge and contributions. An effective group leader encourages team members to research aspects of the joint work in which they have particular knowledge. These employees can then serve as "support" leaders within the team for that work area. If the designated leader seems defensive about his or her authority and reluctant to delegate it, the consultant might emphasize the importance of membership buy-in through their active involvement in researching a problem area and suggesting solutions.

When a leader is particularly inflexible, passive, or defensive, the group tends to take a regressive pathway. Occasionally, however, a group member with natural leadership skills[170] may quietly become an "alternate leader" whom the group trusts and follows. This individual may guide the group toward productive work despite the nominal leader's weaknesses or rigidity. Consultants facing such a situation should try when possible to quietly support this development.

In the research study mentioned earlier, co-author Rudden assessed videotapes of 18 work groups at Maimonides both qualitatively and quantitatively and found striking results about group leaders' effectiveness and the value of alternate leaders in supporting the groups' work.[171]

In a quantitative analysis of groups' performance, it became clear that in groups whose nominal leader struggled to help the team to focus but in which an effective alternate leader emerged, such teams performed successfully: "This may support the idea that when groups are free to influence their leadership, as in more democratic settings, long-range tasks requiring group cooperation may be more likely to be successfully completed. Qualitative observations, too, suggested that in groups in which there were skirmishes witnessed over the leadership with no consistent alternate leader emerging ... the work did suffer."[172]

Katy Steward, an assistant director in Leadership Development at Britain's King's Fund, also emphasizes this concept: "It is not simply the number or quality of individual leaders that determine organizational performance, but the ability of formal and informal leaders to pull together in support of the organization's goals."[173]

To reprise, leaders may need a consultant's help to discern when a group is experiencing a regression because it has encountered obstacles to work, such as unclear goals or a lack of resources, which can then be directly addressed. The consultant can also help a leader to listen to the useful messages that a dissenting subgroup is bearing and to address them, so that the subgroup leaders do not hijack the team's task focus. We have discussed strategies for directing and reinforcing groups' regressive energies and have also addressed the value of recognizing and cultivating support leaders for individual tasks. Designated leaders who can welcome the "natural" leaders within their group to work in synchrony with them—usually by delegating important tasks to them—help their group to become optimally effective. *Such practices form the underpinning for genuine collaborative leadership.*

Addressing Hierarchies and Cultural/Ethnic Differences

The first phase of the Labor-Management Partnership at Maimonides Medical Center accomplished a good deal of effective work. However, it was noted that on a few units, seemingly good solutions to clinical care problems were not maintained six months after their implementation. Lazes reviewed the work of these groups and discovered that several of their members who were lowest in the hospital hierarchy, nurses' aides and licensed practical nurses, had felt inhibited about sharing their ideas. Their experience—accurate or not—was that their contributions, when they struggled to offer them, were neither valued nor incorporated into project results. Their interest in the work waned, and they did not ultimately feel wedded to implementing the group's solutions.

In approaching the next LMP project, on hospital cleanliness, Lazes and a talented union executive vice president, Bruce Richard, discussed how to prevent such a sense of inhibition, exclusion, and disenfranchisement from recurring, especially since many considered environmental service workers to be at the bottom of the hospital hierarchy: "the guys who clean up our mess." Lazes and Richard concluded that preparatory work with the Environmental Services staff might create a safe space in which to help them build the self-confidence to assert themselves later with the professional and managerial staff. In addition, because the Environmental Services Department hired entry-level workers, and thus included many new immigrants from a range of ethnic backgrounds, they felt it important to afford the workers "a chance to express and understand some of their ethnic and racial differences about methods of communication, boundaries (for example, in the amount of eye contact or kind of body language they could comfortably employ), and different ways of expressing their work ethic."[174] These meetings began with Richard revealing his own life experiences about power and disenfranchisement and how he learned to move past a deep sense of inferiority. For many workers, "these discussions were quite illuminating, affording them the time to understand some of the similarities and differences in orientation that each person brought to their work."[175]

After this preparation, the work group began to cohere and decided to themselves solve central problems impeding hospital cleanliness with only one manager pre sent. This group eventually arrived at a number of successful solutions, which included the following:

- Creating a process to ensure that supplies and equipment would be available at the beginning of shifts
- Ensuring that shift-to-shift communications take place to inform workers on the incoming shift about where they need to concentrate
- Creating self-managing work groups
- Purchasing new equipment essential to high-quality cleaning of patient rooms and public areas
- Developing practical methods to monitor hospital cleanliness

Satisfied with their work, they brought their proposals to other co-workers in their department and to senior management. All of their proposals were accepted.

The team was gratified to see the respect with which their work was met and became dedicated to ensuring the success of their plan.

We encourage organizations that contain multiple ethnic groups, who may not always understand each other's culture and communication styles, to undertake such preparatory work. This carries particular importance when the unit groups contain members from different ends of the organizational hierarchy. In that instance, the group leader should receive training in cultural sensitivity and understand the importance of ensuring that each member is encouraged to participate and is made comfortable doing so.

Summary

In this chapter, we argue for the use of both socio-technical and group psychodynamic models for structuring and supporting teams. Each model endorses processes that benefit group cohesion and task performance: the establishment of clear, workable goals, the provision of support for leaders and the engagement of all members' participation.

Without these processes, the pressure to find ways to belong, to be heard, and to be effective can intensify among members, disrupting their work in characteristic ways. The group might implode through in-fighting or attacking outsiders, or through relying excessively on their leader for answers. Alternatively, they might flee into an unrealistic optimism about their work, or may adopt rigid, clichéd thinking that limits their creativity.

The chapter suggests methods by which leaders can speak to the "mood" of their groups when they become distracted from their work in one of these characteristic ways. This can be done by acknowledging the current mood, briefly joining with it, and then playfully or directly shifting the group back to a cooperative work focus.

Leaders should also employ a stance of active listening to all contributions, including dissenting ones, and use conflict resolution techniques to discover workable compromises. They can also recognize when their group has descended into using jargon and cliché, suggesting "unpacking" ideas that seem too rigid or concrete.

Internal consultants can assist leaders whose groups have come to an impasse by reviewing their members' understanding of their central task and of their ability as a team to execute it. This may lead to their helping to restructure the current schedule, or offering more avenues of support. They can also encourage the leader's active cultivation of project leaders for aspects the overall task.

Finally, this chapter addresses how to overcome obstacles that pre sent when groups contain members who occupy different places in the organizational hierarchy, or when members have limited understanding of each others' experiences and cultural expectations.

CHAPTER 6

Union-Driven Innovations

> If you are not at the table, you're on the menu.
>
> *—Lee Saunders, president of the American Federation of State, County, and Municipal Employees, White House conference on "Worker Voice," January 26, 2016*

Labor unions in the United States have contributed powerfully to improving wages, working conditions, and the health and safety of workers. They have ended the soul-killing practice of child labor and have protected workers' rights to fair evaluation and termination procedures. They have saved jobs and at times have initiated changes in organizational systems that made work processes more effective and more meaningful. It is difficult to overestimate the contributions of labor unions to American life.[176]

On the other hand, unions—with their survival under attack for the last several decades—have sometimes succumbed to the bane of all organizations: the concretization and ritualization of their ways of thinking and working. This has afflicted both union groups *and* the management/administration in some sites where we have worked. When two groups in conflict become entrenched and inflexible in their positions, they often drive each other further into maladaptive practices. As this occurs, managers may overlook unions' vital contributions to the American middle class—and thus to the stability of our nation—and may see them merely as enemies who demand unaffordable salaries and block innovative work practices.[177] Conversely, some union officers may deride managers' efforts to seek workers' input into certain strategic decisions as "empty attempts at co-optation."[178] In this chapter, we try to look beyond such polarization to demonstrate the benefit that joint work, and particularly active Labor-Management Partnerships, can provide to unions and to managers/ administrators, especially within healthcare organizations.

Union membership was fairly robust in the 1950s, when over 35 percent of the workforce was unionized. Since the 1960s, however, unions have under gone a steady decline, attacked by federal and state legislators as well as by corporate litigators intent on increasing profits by lowering wages and by thwarting union work rules. By the mid-1960s, union membership had fallen to just over 20 percent of the workforce. Now, as corporations outsource work to poorer nations where wages and safety standards are minimal and unions rare or non ex is tent, American labor unions represent barely 10.7 percent of American workers.[179] Finally, the new corporate emphasis on hiring parttime and contingent workers makes organizing workers much more difficult.[180]

As if these pressures were not enough, in 2018 the Supreme Court created new burdens for unions, mandating them to represent all workers in an organization even if not all employees pay union dues or fees. The ruling overturned the practice of dues deduction from employees' paychecks when unions had negotiated their wages and working conditions.[181] As a result, public sector employees must now indicate to their employer whether or not they want union dues deducted. This new practice has greatly reduced unions' income.

The increasing, often enforced, marginalization of labor unions has put them on the defensive, struggling to organize new members while protecting their basic rights and benefits. Needing to focus on survival, many union leaders stick to their traditional roles of negotiating and enforcing collective bargaining agreements. Labor activists, however, contend that this is a dated approach.[182] Activists feel that to stay viable, unions must directly address the significant changes in the workplace caused by technology, and must share in developing new work systems that enhance job satisfaction and contribute to the survival of the organizations for which their members work while also representing the rights of workers.[183]

One such leader is David Rolf, former president of SEIU 775 in the Pacific Northwest, who contends that unions must adopt innovative strategies such as codetermination (in which workers have the right to vote for representation on a company's board of directors),[184] a common practice in Europe; worker ownership;[185] and Labor-Management Partnerships in order to add value to their organizations and the general economy. Healthcare unions may attract new members—and accrue power within their organizations—by giving frontline staff a voice in decision making about how they can best care for their patients.[186] It has been shown that healthcare unions that do so simultaneously attract new members, improve patient care, and advocate for social justice.[187]

Unlike in industry, about 20 percent of healthcare workers belong to unions, including doctors and nurses. This makes healthcare organizations an important sector in which to focus union energies. Healthcare is also predicted to produce more jobs than any other part of the economy until 2026.[188] Further, frontline staff can directly affect the quality of patient care and patient satisfaction: factors contributing to how current healthcare delivery systems are reimbursed. Healthcare unions can address this potential source of power by encouraging hospitals to undertake employee participation projects such as Labor-Management Partnerships that improve care. Such projects can in turn reconnect frontline staff members to their union leaders, seeing them as more than negotiators for their salaries and benefits. As labor organizer Sidney Hillman stated during World War II,

> Certainly, I believe in collaborating with the employers! That is what unions are for. I even believe in helping an employer function more productively. For then, we will have a claim to higher wages, shorter hours, and greater participation in the benefits of running a smooth industrial machine.[189]

Although Hillman and other union leaders have embraced the strategy of partnership between labor and management, some union leaders view worker participation activities as undermining needed militance, bringing the worker too close to management, where he or she can be co-opted.[190] These union leaders consider that "helping to improve the efficiency of an organization is the job of management, not the union."[191] Yet, working in partnership does not mean erasing the differences in perspectives and goals between labor and management. In participating in a Labor-Management Partnership, unions do not surrender their ability to leverage the use of strikes, protests, walkouts, or community and political pressure to force management's attention when problems affect their members. They might even use these tactics as a means to get management to the table to create a joint process on issues critical to their members and to patients.

Recently, for example, the Vermont Federation of Nurses and Health Professionals, a local of the American Federation of Teachers union, conducted a two-day strike at the University of Vermont Medical Center to induce management to accept a joint process for setting staffing levels.[192] This strike, initiated over working conditions rather than salary, resulted in a robust process that created reasonable, responsible staffing levels for all hospital units and outpatient clinics.[193] Before the strike, management was unwilling to listen to frontline concerns about staffing levels.

There will always be times when union and management leaders disagree on wages, benefits, political activities, and changes in job responsibilities. Such disagreements should not affect the value of joint work for improving patient care, nor should either party hesitate to exercise its responsibility to disagree on matters it deems important.[194] Unions will always need to fight for what they believe is best for their members,[195] and management needs to monitor cost, operational, and legal issues. It is important for them to address their differences, in order to at least clarify divergent perspectives.[196]

Unions, local and national, have employed varied strategies to support joint work. We highlight Labor-Management Partnerships in healthcare organizations, but their fundamental strategies can benefit unions in other economic sectors as well. The main strategies include the following:

1. Creating a consensus within the union about the value or risks of adopting a partnership or

engaging in other types of joint work with management.

2. Clarifying union goals for such activities: What do the members want to gain from joint involvement?
3. Creating research initiatives to examine the potential use of a Partnership process and its impact on union membership.
4. Building the capacity of local unions to support Partnership work.
5. Obtaining support from national unions for Partnership work.

Creating Consensus about Partnership Work within the Local Union

It is critical for local unions to conduct internal conversations about the value of Partnership work with their staff and national union before meeting with management to explore initiation of such activities. Discussions with the national union can create a foundation of support for the local's efforts, helping the local to understand exactly how much their national leaders can contribute in influence, advice, educational materials, and research assistance.

Whether or not a national union has considered supporting Partnerships, the local union will need to discuss with its own leaders and activists, and those in the national union, why Partnership activities might help to solve care-delivery problems that directly and daily affect their members' work.

Internal discussions within a local union can be helpful to consider exploring why and how members might contribute to changing the nature of patient care, and hence their jobs. Union leaders, activists, and frontline care staff have seen firsthand that top-down solutions have not significantly improved patient care outcomes. Recent research studies confirm these observations.[197] Such approaches have certainly not benefited workers, as they often tend to involve onerous staffing schedules and an overriding focus on the bottom line, rather than finding new ways to care for patients.[198]

Initial internal discussions within union locals offer space for thoughtful conversations about why it might be important to work in tandem with management and with other unions, if several unions are involved in a hospital or healthcare delivery system. It is worth exploring what it will mean for union staff, officers, and frontline staff to adapt to a Partnership process. In such a process, the union will need to move away from a predominately adversarial relationship with management to working with management while maintaining separate views and concerns: they will need to learn "to both dance and box at the same time."[199] Union leaders and activists should take the time to reflect on what it means to take responsibility for decisions, rather than allowing management to make mistakes and then take all the blame. These internal, reflective conversations give union leaders time to share their views without getting too far ahead of members. As discussed in the previous chapter, union leaders need the support of their members and staff to sustain the work of a Partnership process without sabotage.

If there is significant resistance to or misunderstanding among union members about working collaboratively, the local leadership might find it helpful to conduct one-on-one conversations with members who have concerns about the new process before launching a Labor-Management Partnership. It is often useful to invite leaders from unions who have already engaged in Partnerships to meet with the local union so that local members can learn about the results of an effective Partnership process. This exchange enables members and leaders to explore the benefits and risks of the process before committing to it.

For some organizations with years of adversarial interactions with managers/administrators, union leaders and members will need to see management demonstrate good faith that they are committing to a nonhierarchical, transactional process. A useful example of how a local union engaged in effective internal conversations about the value of a Labor-Management Partnership took place in Los Angeles with SEIU 721. As described in chapter 3, in late 2012, senior union leaders, shop stewards and rank-and-file members conducted several internal work sessions to discuss forming a Labor-Management

Partnership with the new director of the county's health system. The union used these work sessions to craft an approach to management that would challenge its past record with labor and to gain assurances that this would change. They further examined how the process might achieve their own union-building objectives while improving patient care and access. The local's senior leaders envisioned that Partnership activities would better connect them to member concerns about their work lives. The Partnership process was seen as allowing the union to give frontline staff something new and important to them: a real voice in decisions about improving patient care and their own working conditions.[200]

Clarifying Union Goals for Partnership Work

Along with conversations at the national and local levels about how a Labor-Management Partnership might benefit the union, local unions must create specific goals for working in Partnership. Some past LMP activities have failed because the involved unions did not develop or articulate these.[201] These will be discussed in chapter 8.

The questions that unions need to consider are as follows:

1. What do we need and expect to gain from a Partnership process with management?

2. How can we directly link Partnership goals to the interests of the union and its members?
3. How can we use Partnership activities to improve patient care and safety?
4. Which elements of a Partnership contract should be lobbied for, in order to provide our members with greater opportunities for training?
5. How might our members derive more meaningful work from a Labor-Management Partnership process?
6. How can our involvement in Partnership activities enable us to organize new members to join our union?
7. How can we encourage employers to make it easier for staff to join the union—e.g., through allowing card checks and promising not to undermine union organizing efforts?
8. How can we clarify to staff that Partnership activities were a direct result of the union's negotiating this arrangement?

Clarifying union goals by addressing these questions can help a local union to decide whether it will be worthwhile investing time and funds to support a Partnership.[202]

Common goals that healthcare unions have established for Labor-Management Partnerships include:

- Establishing more direct communication with members by routinely attending problem-solving team meetings, by helping to conduct Partnership training sessions, by conducting meetings in which teams share how they approached their work and their solutions, and by highlighting the work of teams in various newsletters and blogs
- Providing members with time apart from their daily work to address patient care issues and to reduce work-arounds[203]
- Devising ways to improve patient satisfaction and staff and patient safety
- Creating opportunities for frontline staff to weigh in on new purchases of equipment and supplies
- Developing training programs to enable employees to master the new skills that might result from the restructuring efforts
- Shifting labor relations from an adversarial to a problem-solving process based on mutual interests
- Creating more meaningful work
- Increasing union membership by creating new jobs and by having workers who are not in the union join the union

Both qualitative and quantitative research methods can be used to track the achievement of such goals.

As an example of this process, the six specific union-building goals adopted by SEIU 1199 at Maimonides Medical Center were (1) to deepen communication and engagement with members; (2) to improve labor relations problems and reduce arbitrations; (3) to increase members' contributions to political action activities (to a union PAC fund); (4) to improve attendance at political rallies that support state and city funding for Maimonides and for political candidates who endorse workers' rights and social justice issues; (5) to increase communication within the hospital about the Partnership process and the union's role in it; and (6) to recruit more employees to join the union.[204]

These union goals were eventually incorporated into the overall goals of the Maimonides Medical Center's Labor-Management Strategic Alliance.[205] These goals were tracked quarterly, and major improvements occurred in all areas.[206]

Union Building Outcomes SEIU 1199/Maimonides

Attendance at political rallies: Increased by 48 percent
Arbitrations: Reduced by 64 percent
New shop stewards: Increased by 265 percent
Political action contributions: Increased by 45 percent
Union membership: Increased by 18 percent

Research Initiatives

Getting involved in Partnership activities will require healthcare unions to broaden their research activities. One shift will require unions and their members to assist in conducting research to document the extent to which Partnership activities improve patient care and create more meaningful jobs. This is quite important since often this documentation doesn't take place.

Unions should also consider conducting, in the future, their own research on delivery system issues and trends, as hospital administrators tend not to share their research findings about such matters with labor leaders lest their data be used against them.[207] Such research is quite important in order to make strategic decisions about where to deploy resources for Partnership activities. It turns out that unions are often in a better position than management to collect this sector data, as they have access to information from a broad range of healthcare systems.

As healthcare organizations continue to increase the use of various technologies and have access, to some extent, to a global workforce (even within the healthcare sector), U.S. healthcare unions would also benefit from expanding the scope of their research to include understanding how new technologies will impact future jobs. Having this information will help union leaders prepare members for these jobs and have sufficient time to organize needed trainings.

Whereas many local unions have not conducted such research, national unions often have funds for, and experience with, these investigations. National unions that represent healthcare workers, such as the American Federation of Teachers, the Committee of Interns and Residents, the Doctors Council, and the Service Employees International Union have assigned staff to research the areas cited previously. Some larger healthcare locals, such as SEIU 721 in Los Angeles, SEIU 1199 in New York City, and SEIU Healthcare Pennsylvania, have allocated funds for this nontraditional union research.

This expanded research approach is a significant departure from current union research priorities that focus, for the most part, on preparing for contract negotiations and helping to structure new organizing campaigns.[208] By expanding research activities, U.S. healthcare unions can ensure that Labor-Management Partnerships focus on the most important issues.[209]

Building the Capacity of Local Unions to Support Partnership Work

When a hospital or delivery system begins a Labor-Management Partnership process, or another approach using frontline staff input to improve patient care, they frequently reassign staff to manage the new initiative. They also generally hire experienced consultants to advise about approaches that have succeeded in similarly structured organizations. Unions should ensure that this occurs and should make similar reassignments, as well as considering whether or not to hire their own consultant.

Because Partnership activities often result in changes in delivery system processes, and sometimes even staffing changes, healthcare unions (local and national) must determine the best way to become full partners in guiding the process, particularly in educating the workforce to handle the resultant work changes. Again, to actively participate in the Labor-Management Partnership with the Los Angeles County Department of Health Services, the president of the local union assigned a key senior adviser, Patricia Castillo, to work part-time at developing the Partnership process.

After two years of productive Partnership activities, it became apparent to union leaders that the local needed to strengthen its capacity to keep up with and sometimes to initiate joint projects. After considering different paths forward, they decided that Castillo should be freed to work full-time on the Partnership. Two research staff members were also assigned to work with her to support the work teams as they set about their increasingly complex tasks. With these resources, Castillo could work more closely with the union's shop stewards and with hospital and clinic staff to continue building enthusiasm and support for Partnership activities. CEO Katz also agreed to relieve county employees from their full-time jobs to work with Castillo as Healthcare Transformation Advocates (internal consultants and mentors). As of 2020, there are now 17 such Advocates. The county has paid their salaries, while the union has funded Castillo and her assigned staff.

SEIU 721 found that reassigning their own staff and creating Healthcare Transformation Advocate jobs has enabled them to become an active partner with the County Department of Health Services in the joint work. Investing in these personnel changes made the union ambidextrous, working on partnership matters in addition to traditional union activities. However, they have discovered challenges to sustaining this new role. "Working sometimes jointly and sometimes separately with management is not an easy process after a history of fighting tooth and nail with the county administration. Nevertheless, it has become a crucial strategy for our union to get stronger and to grow. We have worked very hard to make this transition,"[210] stated Castillo.

Like SEIU 721, other locals have decided to make staff changes to work more fully in partnership processes. These locals include the Committee of Interns and Residents (CIR),[211] the Doctors Council,[212] and SEIU Healthcare Pennsylvania.[213] They have concluded that broadening their capacity for partnership work by hiring new staff members enabled them to become more effective in improving patient care and in advancing their union-building initiatives.[214]

At Kaiser Permanente, the Coalition of Unions, which initially represented most of the locals within Kaiser,[215] has taken a different approach to supporting partnership activities. Although union leaders from each local are members of the Kaiser Partnership process, most staff who work on Partnership initiatives are hired by the Coalition of Kaiser Permanente Unions itself: local unions have not for the most part reassigned internal staff. There are benefits and risks to this approach. Because the participating locals in the Coalition had little need to reassign staff to new roles and responsibilities, they did not need to train them in the new skills crucial to do this work. Instead, funds from these local unions contribute to the Coalition of Kaiser Permanente Unions' hiring staff for Partnership projects. This saves locals time and effort, but since they have not incorporated Partnership activities as a core practice for themselves, they have not developed the relationships with the employees working on these projects that win their loyalty and grow local membership.[216]

Support from National Unions for Partnership Work

Although most Labor-Management Partnerships are established at the local level, several national unions have supported these activities.[217] The Amalgamated and Textile Workers Union (ACTWU), American Federation of Teachers (AFT), Service Employees International Union (SEIU), and United Auto Workers (UAW) have all invested in Labor-Management Partnerships, each employing different methods.

The ACTWU established an Industrial Research department. Its research helped ACTWU locals anticipate and prepare for changes in the textile and garment industries and led the national union to propose the Partnership processes at the Hathaway shirt company, Levi Strauss, Hickey Freeman, and others, which created new modular manufacturing systems. Hundreds of jobs were saved in assembly plants and distribution centers as a result. The ACTWU provided funds to local unions to educate their members about the changes affecting their manufacturing sector. It has also funded union-friendly partnership consultants to establish and consult to Partnerships.

The American Federation of Teachers' Division for Nurses and Health Professionals established a Learning Collaborative in 2016 to accelerate joint activities between AFT local frontline staff and management counter parts.[218] The Collaborative attempts to bring together labor and management safety committees from different hospitals on a yearly basis to study effective practices for ensuring staff and patient safety. The workshops feature a highly interactive process between union and management representatives and have resulted in several successful new endeavors by participants.

SEIU's Healthcare Division has established yet another approach to encourage Labor-Management Partnerships. Dr. Toni Lewis, a recent director of this division, began to convene quarterly meetings with several of the larger SEIU locals representing healthcare workers to expose them to the experiences of workers who have already adopted LMPs in their hospital systems. The Healthcare Division funded three Labor-Management Partnership projects, in the Los Angeles County Department of Health Services, Cook County Hospital in Chicago, and Allegheny Medical Center in Pittsburgh. Dr. Lewis retained Cornell's Healthcare Transformation project[219] consultants, including co-author Lazes, to provide education, research, and additional consultants to support the new LMPs.

We have already described the first site funded by SEIU, the LA-DHS Labor-Management Partnership. At Cook County Hospital in Chicago, the funds were used for an intervention focused on enabling labor and management, who had a history of considerable friction and mistrust, to collaborate better. It was hoped that an outside consultant could encourage labor and management leaders to find areas for joint work. To this end, an initial Labor-Management project at Cook County focused on reducing wait times in the outpatient clinic and on expediting the scheduling of specialty care appointments. Results of this effort are discussed in chapter 8.

The third Labor-Management Partnership process funded by SEIU was at Allegheny General Hospital. The focus of their Partnership activities has been establishing unit-based teams on all inpatient units to improve patient care and safety and reduce costs. Nurses constituted the initial team members, as SEIU represented only the nurses at Allegheny. Their work produced significant improvements in patient and staff safety discussed later. Unit-based work continues at Allegheny General Hospital.

Beyond providing funds to support the three Partnership projects, Lewis used national union leadership meetings, SEIU board meetings, and several meetings of their national Healthcare Quality Advisory Committee to broadcast the experiences of these Partnerships. Her vision has been to encourage locals to establish similar activities, learning from what has worked and what has not in these sites.

National unions can be useful in encouraging, or even pressuring, health systems administrators to establish Labor-Management Partnerships. This assistance might be extremely helpful when a local union cannot marshal enough pressure on the administration themselves.

Summary

Union leaders are acutely aware that their membership is declining because of widespread antiunion laws and corporate practices, particularly the ongoing practice of moving jobs offshore. They understand the need to do things differently in order to keep their mission alive.

Unions in all economic sectors still need to represent workers when their rights are ignored or abused. Several national unions have now articulated, however, that it is also important to involve frontline staff in efforts to improve manufacturing processes or patient care practices. As Bruce Richard of SEIU 1199 states, "Being extremely proactive is much more critical now for unions than it was in the past. New and innovative approaches must be adopted to protect the jobs and wages of workers. Traditional approaches are no longer sufficient."[220]

Healthcare organizations are currently undergoing drastic changes as they try to better coordinate and integrate care systems, use new technologies, and respond to different reimbursement arrangements. Such systemic shifts will result in significant job changes: eliminating some, creating others. In the past, redesigning services, creating new jobs, and finding ways to improve patient care rested solely in the hands of management. Creating comprehensive healthcare Labor-Management Partnerships enables unions and frontline staff to be included in the design of new delivery systems that they can ensure will be patient and worker-centered. In addition, establishing Partnerships expands the ability of employees to work in a safe environment in which they are able to raise problems without fearing reprisals.[221]

A new development initiated by SEIU 721 in Los Angeles County offers an additional benefit for unions who participate in Labor Management Partnerships. A system-wide process focused on creating a "just culture" in all county healthcare facilities encourages staff to report to management, without retaliation, any errors, near-miss events, adverse events, or unsafe conditions with these facilities.[222] This new system has helped employees to report mistakes without fear of reprisal and allows the LMP to access important data about clinical care practice.

To summarize the benefits to unions of joint labor-management activities, Fran Todd, a nurse practitioner involved in the LA-DHS Partnership, observed, "These activities have mobilized significant numbers of members, who now see their union as providing them opportunities to have a voice in decision-making and in improving patient care."[223] Todd stressed that "many new union activists were not interested in the traditional work of the union, but once worker participation became a priority for our local, they saw the benefit of being part of this process."[224] David Rolf and other union leaders have agreed: "Unions need to change if the labor movement is to thrive again and workers are to find greater dignity at work."[225]

PART THREE

The Future

CHAPTER 7

Future Approaches for Labor-Management Partnerships

> Insanity is doing the same thing over and over again and expecting different results.
>
> —*Albert Einstein*

As Lazes wrote earlier, my journey to improve patient care systems began in Newark during the 1970s when I was alarmed by the disjointed and inferior care that patients were receiving at Martland Hospital. Dr. Rudden experienced similar dismay while training at Bellevue Hospital in the early '70s. Sadly, similar problems persist today in most communities. Patients still face long waits to see care providers. Many have difficulty obtaining appointments with specialists. There is often limited follow-up and support available to patients with complex conditions or behavioral health issues that require ongoing care and monitoring. Patients with chronic health problems, in particular, remain underserved by our healthcare systems. Many insurance plans, further, do not commonly pay for preventive measures even though these would yield long-term cost savings as well as better health. Over 8.5 percent of Americans—27.5 million people—still lack any health insurance[226] and must seek care in emergency rooms when they require medical help. This is not just an inner-city problem, but a national crisis.[227] Our systems of delivering comprehensive care are broken.[228]

In the preceding chapters, we have discussed the fact that most state and federal approaches to the healthcare crisis primarily seek to increase access to insurance coverage and to cut costs but do not address many of the deepest flaws in our healthcare systems. We have offered practical approaches for initiating and expanding Labor-Management Partnerships in our medical centers to tap the knowledge of frontline staff in a cooperative, organized manner in partnership with management. This approach can improve individual care systems, often increasing job satisfaction while simultaneously cutting costs. We have shown specific ways in which collaborative leadership grants all stakeholders a voice in crafting systemic changes. We have cautioned that creating extensive organizational changes is a complex and time-consuming process:[229] staff, unions, and managers need time to accept, to learn how to engage together in an LMP process, and to envision its expansion to tackle system-wide issues. We now explore additional innovative processes that, along with Labor-Management Partnerships, have transformed current care practices to offer new methods for delivering more coherent, accessible, and integrated care.

The Worker Lab

The Worker Lab was created by David Rolf, the dynamic former president of SEIU 775, in Seattle, Washington, in 2014. He developed this initiative to encourage workers, regardless of where they are employed, to identify methods of improving existing services or creating new systems and products. The Worker Lab resembles the Danish Employee-Driven Innovation initiatives (EDI) described in chapter 2 and was informed by the work of Silicon Valley entrepreneurs. It provides a worker or a small group of workers with start-up funds (upward of $150,000) to develop their ideas for new products or services. Project ideas can come from SEIU 775 members or from any other worker who has learned about this resource.

Potential projects are submitted to the Lab's advisory board, which chooses which proposals to support. Once a project is selected, consultants are assigned to assist each project leader in refining the idea and in examining its feasibility. The Worker Lab provides additional consultants to assist in developing business plans and in securing more funds to test the viability of the new product or service. Periodically, the Worker Lab brings together the leaders of recently funded projects to share their experiences and thus maximize their learning about starting up a small business or services.[230]

The Lab solicits ideas for projects annually. Financial support for its work comes from several progressive foundations, entrepreneurs, and the SEIU. Describing his inspiration for the Lab, Rolf explained, "The use of innovative strategies has been critical for Silicon Valley companies to be successful. We have tried to adopt this strategy to help our labor movement benefit from the creative ideas of frontline staff. We know that some ideas won't be successful, but through this process of creating new systems and products, we are certain to fund some important breakthroughs. This why we see the Worker Lab as so important."[231] Rolf views the creation of such new products and services as benefiting the labor movement by expanding our economy and creating new jobs. For Rolf, the Worker Lab is part of a larger national strategy to reposition unions so that they can grow and remain an important force for social justice.

Although the approach of the Worker Lab is not currently part of the repertory of most healthcare Labor-Management Partnerships, it could become an extremely important means for soliciting and supporting creative ideas from frontline staff who are already focused on patient-care improvement projects. When this approach was implemented in Denmark via the Employee-Driven Innovation initiatives, numerous ideas from frontline staff resulted in making it easier for patients to access care and receive treatment at home. An early example from the United States of a frontline worker contributing her ideas toward a striking and highly profitable new invention is that of Lupe Hernandez, a student nurse from Bakersfield, California, who invented the hand sanitizer in 1966. Hernandez observed that sanitation was a considerable problem for people with no immediate access to soap and water and realized that putting alcohol into gel form would provide similar or even better protection. This nurse called in her idea to an inventions hotline and the product was developed.[232] A National Healthcare Labor-Management Partnership Workers Lab could achieve similar outcomes. Such a dedicated effort, along with newly developed processes or technologies, could generate new revenue streams for hospitals and community health centers.

Technology Innovation Centers

A second approach to creating healthcare delivery system breakthroughs would be for a group of healthcare Labor-Management Partnerships to *directly* support expansion in the use of existing technologies and in the development of new ones. New, more user-friendly technologies, from improved robotics for surgery, to devices for self-monitoring the progress of an illness or a patient's response to treatment, to new equipment to support home care, to smart cards enabling patients and providers to quickly access a patient's history, medications, test results, and contact details can all help control healthcare costs and improve patient outcomes.

In the 1960s and 1970s, a brilliant and innovative engineer, Mike Cooley, known as a scientist with shop-floor credentials, pioneered an innovative way to use existing and new technologies in industry. Working at the Lucas Aerospace Company in England, Cooley became distressed by the almost yearly cyclical downturns that occurred there, causing workers to be laid off for extended periods of time. After observing these downturns for several years, Cooley and some of his trade union colleagues decided to find a way to avoid the layoffs and benefit the communities where they lived. After discussions within the union, with municipal leaders in London, and with academics, Cooley and his colleagues obtained funding to create community-based technology development centers in the neighborhoods surrounding Lucas. These centers developed prototypes and then manufactured products that made profits, hiring Lucas workers to produce them during cyclical downturns. Lucas workers stipulated that the products be not only profitable but socially and environmentally responsible.[233] These centers eventually became part of the Greater London Enterprise Board (GLEB), a citywide economic development organization that enabled the centers to operate all year.

The British Technology Development Centers served as industrial incubators, similar to the Worker Lab, but emphasized current and new technologies. Staffing the centers were Lucas workers, university faculty, and student experts in production methods and new technologies. Within two years, the centers developed more than 150 new products such as electric bikes, small-scale wind turbines, energy conservation services, devices for individuals with various disabilities, children's play equipment, and community computer networks. The Technology Development Centers established training programs for Lucas workers to learn new skills so that they could easily obtain such jobs during downturns. Cooley's creativity harnessed the knowledge and skills of frontline workers to maintain full employment.[234]

Although hospital and health systems do not have cyclical downturns, creating technology incubators sponsored by a group of healthcare Labor-Management Partnerships is well worth considering. New self-or home-monitoring devices can avert medical crises, reducing costly emergency room visits and hospitalizations.

Currently, U.S. equipment manufacturers are the primary investors in research and development for new medical devices. These companies lack regular access to the knowledge, ideas, and skills of frontline staff aside from the physicians they hire as consultants; hence their devices are not always user-friendly. These manufacturers retain all profits from new inventions. The experience of the Lucas aerospace workers thus poses an alternative process, in which frontline healthcare workers directly contribute to enhancing current technologies and developing new ones. Supported by healthcare Partnerships, this approach might provide new income streams while ensuring that the new technologies are used to expand rather than eliminate jobs.[235]

Funding for healthcare technology incubators and expanding the Worker Lab approach might stem from hospital research and development bud gets, foundation grants, the national unions representing healthcare workers, private foundations, and state and federal bud gets. A portion of revenues from new products might be funneled back into healthcare incubators to cover future research and development costs. Employee Driven Innovation funding in Denmark has come from national unions, hospitals and health departments, and the federal government. Universities might provide another source of support for these initiatives. In the past, student and faculty at academic centers played important roles in helping several manufacturing companies reduce costs, create new products, and save jobs.[236]

Accelerating the Creation of New Healthcare Delivery Systems

Although many healthcare Labor-Management Partnerships will continue to focus on incremental change, future LMPs should also use interventions to promote significant breakthroughs for providing more integrated, high-quality, affordable care. Practitioners such as Stu Winby, president of Spring Network, argue that "only by more radical and transformative activities[237] will we be able to create healthcare delivery systems that provide better outcomes."[238] A practical method to speed the process of transforming healthcare delivery systems is Winby's Work Innovation Network (WIN) process, which begins with a large-system intervention. Although there are several kinds of large system interventions,[239] we chose to highlight the WIN approach since it has been conducted within hospital settings and research exists about its composition, process and outcomes.[240] Winby, a consultant trained in clinical psychology, behavioral medicine, and human factor engineering, created and directed Hewlett-Packard's Factory of the Future process from 1989 to 2000. This initiative was established to continue ongoing innovation at HP, which was considered at the time to represent the gold standard in manufacturing.

The WIN process begins with an intensive two-day retreat, a "Decision Accelerator," to which all stakeholders in a healthcare system are invited: administrators, frontline staff, patients, insurers, and community and health department representatives. The latter groups, whom Winby terms "end users," pre sent their unmet care needs or explore new ways of restructuring reimbursements within a redesigned healthcare system. Guests (termed "radicals") from other organizations that have accomplished transformative activities are invited to encourage participants to consider outside-the-box remedies for their systemic shortcomings.[241]

The retreat creates the case for changing the current system by identifying central organizational problem areas and envisioning new structures to correct them, with all stakeholders accorded time and space to offer their input. Action Teams are established during the Decision Accelerator to work on each area identified as requiring change. The teams comprise a cross-section of participants to ensure a broad range of experiences, knowledge, and skills among their membership. Each Action Team is tasked with creating a process or structure to "enhance the patient experience"[242] while better integrating the system. These teams are provided time to analyze their work area and to obtain more detailed feedback about their task from other participants.

Following the retreat, each Action Team meets weekly to set quantifiable goals and to continue designing structures and processes that accord with the overall strategy established during the initial meeting. The teams' work is reviewed by senior organization leaders on a 30-, 60-, and 90-day basis after the retreat. During this working period, teams ideally receive support from internal consultants, which is critical to their functioning. Teams usually require three to four months to complete and submit their new process recommendations ("design specs") to senior management. Once the leadership accepts suggestions for the new processes, Action Team members implement their solutions and submit monthly reports to senior management about their outcomes.

Like Labor-Management Partnership teams, WIN Action Teams work on solutions through an iterative process[243] of devising experiments that test multiple potential solutions in order to finalize an outcome with significant results (see figure 4). Unlike in the LMP process used at Maimonides and LA-DHS, unions have not had a role in helping to design the WIN process, identifying teams once goals are established, and overseeing implementation of solutions by Action Teams. The WIN process is thus management-driven, although it does powerfully engage the thinking and efforts of frontline workers.

WIN is extremely successful because it creates an opportunity for all significant stakeholders in a healthcare delivery system to intensively analyze the current system and collectively identify aspects that require change. The approach enables all participants to picture the issues facing their current system and creates a scenario in which the authority and will to revamp the delivery system is pre sent "in the room."[244] A significant aspect of this large group intervention is that it enables key stakeholders (not only clinical staff of a hospital system but community organization staff, state and federal health department staff involved in reimbursement policies, and insurance company representatives) to meet and exchange ideas from various points of view. One advantage of this large group approach is that it encourages "debate intensity"—which can contribute to the formulation of unique and novel solutions.[245]

Figure 4. Steps in the Work Innovation Network Process

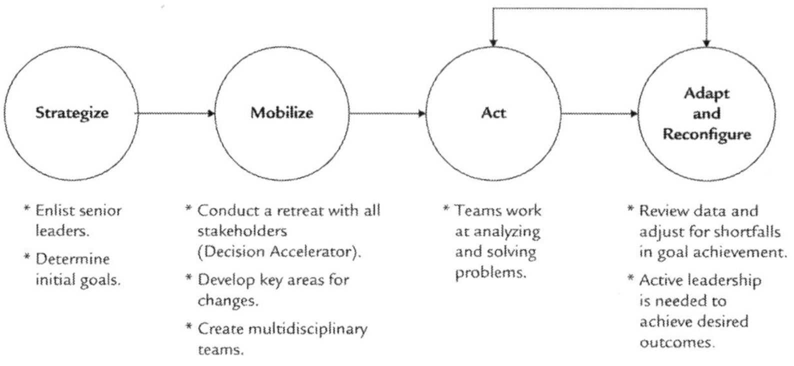

Winby has implemented the WIN process at both Alegent Health (Omaha, Nebraska)[246] and Fairview Health Services (Minneapolis, Minnesota).[247] Each of these systems used traditional inpatient and outpatient silos prior to WIN, with patient care provided in a fairly fragmented fashion. Neither had instituted meaningful relationships with local community health groups. These organizations used the WIN process to successfully transform their delivery systems into Patient-Centered Medical Homes as well as to strengthen specialty services in their delivery systems. Fairview also established care coordinator positions to oversee patients' overall treatment in the care system and in the community. It developed new reimbursement arrangements with Medicare and with several private insurance companies to pay for coordinating patients' care. Creating these new reimbursement agreements was critical to compensating Fairview for the new services they offered and for their loss of revenue due to reduced hospital admissions. "Without 'out of the box' thinking, our delivery systems would still be locked into their older ways of working,"[248] stated Terry Carroll, former senior vice president for transformation, Fairview Health Services.

As healthcare organization leaders continue to explore methods for creating integrated delivery systems, approaches like WIN (a systemic intervention focused on a desired future state) can be helpful. Although WIN has not been applied to current healthcare Labor-Management Partnerships, its approach offers an important method for expanding the repertoire of Labor-Management Partnership activities and complements the values and philosophy of partnership work.

Despite the fact that WIN and similar large group interventions have been successful in launching teams that study patient care problems and suggest cost-control measures, their approach is at times compromised by an uneven power gradient between the teams and the administrators who eventually control all decisions about their work. To address this problem, new approaches have helped to encourage all stakeholders to speak up, although these are implemented only during the initial large group meeting:

1. Opportunities were created for less "powerful" stakeholders to have the time to pull together

their ideas and concerns by themselves. An effective process has been pre-retreat caucusing of these stakeholders.

2. High-powered stakeholders were coached on listening and trying to understand the views of all contributors. This helped to create an atmosphere of freedom for all pre sent, so that they could suggest changes to the current system. It helped to uncover important issues that high-powered senior leaders didn't see.

3. A balanced number of all stakeholders were invited, so that clinical staff and managers at lower levels felt able to speak.[249]

Including Excluded Actors

It is critical that the next phase of Labor-Management Partnerships include patient representatives in the decision-making process for systemic change. Other than the WIN approach, which included patients in the design phase of the change process,[250] patients have been excluded from a direct role in LMP activities. Without their involvement, however, healthcare leaders and frontline staff lack essential information about the impact that the changes they are devising might have on patients' lives.

It would be extremely useful for Action Teams, as they experiment with changes in the care process, to meet with focus groups of the patients whom their units or departments serve. This feedback would have particular value for patients with chronic and complicated health issues, who may have special needs in accessing care, and who often struggle to understand diagnoses and treatment plans devised by multiple, nonconversing specialists. Such patients often need advocates to help understand their intersecting diagnoses, to advise them on monitoring their symptoms, to review multiple medication regimens, and to help navigate the delivery system.[251] Systems that offer more coordinated care will be a boon, but such patients will still likely continue to need care managers.

The Affordable Care Act created funds for "patient navigators," a job similar to patient advocate, on a national level. Sixty-three million dollars were allocated to healthcare systems that made these navigators available to their patients.[252] In practice, however, these jobs have focused only on helping Americans understand their healthcare insurance options so that they can make informed choices about which plan to purchase. Creating patient advocate positions would complement the roles of these patient navigators to ensure that patients benefit from new care systems.

Including patient feedback in planning systems changes is crucial. As many care system departments, such as billing or finance, remain siloed, caregivers often have little information about the larger systemic issues their patients face. *Kaiser Health News* reported in November 2019, for example, that the University of

Virginia Health System had sued 36,000 patients over the course of six years for more than $100 million, "seizing wages and savings and even pushing families into bankruptcy."[253] The news created an uproar for the UVA system's medical and nursing staff, as well as its larger community. Three senior staff members, Drs. Scott Heysell, Rebecca Dillingham, and Michael Williams, wrote a widely circulated letter in response to the report, decrying this practice: "We felt betrayed ... and we had, by extension, betrayed those who had relied on us ... we are outraged. We stand with those that have been financially injured, whose bank accounts have been looted, whose homes have been swallowed as if they were built on quicksand ... all as a result of having sought our care."[254]

Kimberley Acquaviva, a professor of health policy at UVA's nursing school, wrote on Twitter about her discussions in class that this issue "has been painful for them as nurses who care deeply about the patients and families they serve.... As a class, we talked about the power that nurses have to shape the lives of the patients and families by advocating for system change."[255] Without patient input about the full impact of the care system on their lives, however, it is unlikely that LMPs in their current form will address such practices.

By contrast, and with an eye to future goals for our health systems, consider the highly collaborative design process for the new Orbis Medical Center in the

Netherlands: "The overall concept of designing the hospital was to create the best environment for patients: a healing environment with a true human interaction between patients, nurses, doctors and other staff."[256] The design process for this new hospital involved all relevant stakeholders: the Patients' Board, the Workers' Council, the unions. In addition, it incorporated extensive staff member recommendations about creating an environment in which they might work more productively and happily.

The hospital, completed in 2008, features a huge atrium, a food court, comfortable chairs in waiting areas, chairs that convert into beds for family members in patient rooms, and bedside media terminals allowing patients to order meals, watch TV, call nursing staff, and view their chart, including all recent test and procedure results. Smart cards were developed for doctors and nurses, enabling providers to quickly access their patients' history, medications, test results, and information about the patient's outpatient physicians, pharmacists, family contacts, etc. Hospital designs in the United States have incorporated some of these patient-friendly features, which derived from soliciting patients' concerns.

However, Theodora Swenson notes that many hospitals have adopted generic "hotel or airport" designs with the intent to comfort patients without actually doing so: "We need to stop designing hospitals in isolation and first answer the question: What *is* healthcare? Only once we understand the purpose of what we are designing for can we then decide how to build it. We need to understand the ecosystem—the complex infrastructure of healthcare—before we can design hospitals."[257]

To actively consult and incorporate the expressed needs of staff and patients through a collaborative process should be a future goal for our unions, healthcare workers, and administrators.

Summary

In this chapter, we considered strategies that offer the potential for increasing revenue to medical centers while at the same time enlisting the creative and practical ideas of their staff. The Worker Lab, established in Seattle and based on practices used in Silicon Valley, offers encouragement for workers, regardless of where they are employed, to identify methods to improve services or to create new systems and products. The Worker Lab provides a worker or small group of workers with startup funds to develop their ideas. While the Worker Lab focuses primarily on the development of new processes for patient care, we also encourage groups of healthcare Labor Management Partnerships to form Technology Development centers such as the one developed at Lucas Aerospace in England and supported by surrounding universities. The development of new methods for healthcare technology may provide a source of funds for medical centers and their Labor Management Partnerships.

In addition, we discussed intensive large group work sessions that can accelerate the initial work of Strategic Alliances, Labor-Management Partnerships, or new health systems development. A particular methodology based on programs employed in Silicon Valley by Stuart Winby (The Work Innovation Network Process) and used at Alegent and Fairview Medical Centers is described in detail.

Finally, we discussed the need for Labor Management Partnerships to include patient feedback about care access and care provision from the very beginning of their work. Further, clinical staff need to be made aware of their center's approach to patients who are late in paying their bills so that they can ensure that such practices meet the ethical standards of their professions.

CHAPTER 8

Analyzing Value, Preventing Failures

> Success is not final, failure is not fatal, it is the courage to continue that counts.
>
> —*Winston Churchill*

> A society characterized by generalized reciprocity is more efficient than a distrusting society.... If we don't have to balance every exchange instantly, we can get a lot more accomplished.
>
> —*Robert D. Putnam*

We have repeatedly underscored that the development of healthcare Labor-Management Partnerships channeling the knowledge and experience of frontline staff is a highly rewarding process, but one that presents challenges. The challenge for labor involves shifting from an adversarial relationship with management to collaborating to create change in the workplace. An LMP process requires unions to balance working jointly on organizational change strategies with their traditional responsibility to represent workers in conflicts with management. For management, the Partnership process necessitates sharing production, quality, and financial information with staff and unions, and involving them in decisions ranging from purchasing equipment and supplies to designing new care structures and uses of technology. For an organization to fully commit and carry through a successful Labor-Management Partnership, leaders on each side must come to identify the value of this work and commit to it.

A primary value of workers' involvement with decision making in healthcare settings is that, as we have shown, patient care is improved while employees' work lives become enriched and more satisfying. More efficient delivery processes and increased patient satisfaction scores also result in cost savings in several dimensions. What is rarely addressed, however, is that participating in these workplace activities contributes to employees' increased confidence, improved skills, and motivation for contributing to civic life beyond the hospital. The first section of this chapter focuses on this finding, which is of great importance for our society. In the second section, we will provide an analysis of site-specific difficulties encountered while starting or sustaining some Labor-Management Partnership processes, with an eye toward preventing similar problems in the future.

Increasing Civic Participation

The shrinking of civic participation among U.S. citizens has reached alarming proportions. The decline in numbers of citizens voting in national elections provides a startling example of their alienation from a process central to democracy. Only 61 percent of U.S. citizens voted in the 2016 presidential election, the lowest voter turnout since 1996.[258] Further, there is a documented decrease in citizens participating in community organizations. For example, Americans are about half as likely to work for a political party or attend a political rally now as they were in the 1970s. The number of office seekers from school boards to town councils has shrunk by about 15 percent.[259]

In the United States, Ron Putnam, a prominent sociologist and observer of civic life, has documented how civic passivity contributes to a decline in community resources; a lack of public policies to improve education and healthcare, especially for poorer citizens; and a rise in crime.[260] Putnam also argues that declining civic participation in our nation undermines our democracy and perhaps even our political stability.[261]

Scandinavian countries, particularly Norway, have found a direct connection between citizens participating in workplace involvement activities and subsequent engagement in their wider communities. Worker participation activities are viewed there as a vital approach to encouraging civic activism. Norwegians feel that to preserve an active democracy in which citizens can retain individual and collective freedoms, participation in their communities and in their nation is critical.

Political scientist Max Elden and sociologist Bob Karasek have each documented the connection between greater workplace decision making and greater civic participation. Karasek, in seminal research conducted in Sweden based on national aggregate data from 1968 and 1974,[262] demonstrated that workers' "job decision freedom" (the ability to make decisions) and their control over their work pace and job responsibilities directly correlated with their degree of political and civic participation. His studies revealed that workers holding more "passive" jobs that lacked decision making and broad job responsibilities were much less likely to engage in either political or leisure activities.[263] Elden's research, complementing Karasek's, again documents that greater workplace autonomy in self-managing work groups increases workers' civic participation.[264] This synergy clearly seems to reduce civic passivity.[265]

To investigate the connection between workplace and civic participation in the United States, co-author Lazes approached labor and management leaders at Maimonides Medical Center for permission to research this question. Pam Brier, then CEO of Maimonides, and Bruce Richard, executive VP of SEIU 1199, became co-investigators. In addition to their intensive involvement in Labor-Management Partnership activities at Maimonides,[266] both Brier and Richard were extremely interested in whether hospital worker participation influenced their community activism, as both Brier and Richard have for years been directly involved in multiple community endeavors. Over the years of the Maimonides Partnership process, Brier, Richard, and Lazes had each heard anecdotal evidence from frontline staff about their new involvement in various community activities. Was there a real connection between workplace and civic participation, or did frontline staff chosen or electing to participate in Partnership activities already tend to participate in community organizations?

After much discussion, we decided to track two outcomes relevant to community participation that were relatively easy to measure. The first was to assess the degree to which frontline staff participated in political action events (such as rallies and protests supporting state and local funding for the hospital and community health organizations) or volunteered for community work. The second traced whether employees contributed part of their pay, on a regular basis, to support their union's political activities. Anonymous surveys were distributed annually to frontline staff participating in departmental labor-management committees and various work groups from 2002 to 2006.

Over the five years of this study, we found a 48 percent increase in attendance at political rallies and involvement in community work by frontline staff participating in Labor-Management Partnership activities. Contributions to political activities also increased by 45 percent over the five years. These outcomes were particularly noteworthy because SEIU 1199 had already achieved high levels of attendance at political events and had encouraged members to work with community organizations prior to the LMP at Maimonides.

Focus groups of frontline staff participating in Maimonides' LMP process explored this question qualitatively. These groups revealed that employees felt more inclined to participate in civic activities because of the leadership and decision-making skills they had acquired in their work with the LMP. Specifically, many staff members articulated that their opportunity to improve patient care through working as a team[267] made them feel newly respected by both management and their peers.[268] Increased self-confidence from running groups and handling the inevitable conflicts that arose within them was mentioned as contributing significantly to the workers' motivation to apply their skills elsewhere.

Apart from the significant benefits that Labor-Management Partnerships bring to healthcare organizations by reducing costs and solving significant problems in patient care delivery and integration, this civic contribution is vital. During turbulent times in which citizens seem alienated from government and from the essential practices of democracy, it is crucial to discover ways of strengthening their skills and motivation to participate in national and community organizations at every level. As we documented in this chapter and in chapter 2, workplace participation can reduce the feelings of disenfranchisement and helplessness bedeviling many citizens. Strengthening understanding of civic structures and offering opportunities in our schools to assist community groups[269] will help to acquaint future voters with the importance of participation in community and national democratic structures.

As Einar Thorsrud, a key Norwegian scholar of both workplace and civic participation, stated several years ago, "Continuous learning, support between colleagues, and meaningful [work] relations is important to workplace productivity and civil society."[270]

We will now provide an analysis of healthcare Labor-Management Partnerships that did not work—either from the outset, or from some later point—so that frontline workers and managers interested in creating a new Partnership can learn from these failures and avoid their missteps.

Labor-Management Partnerships That Failed: An Analysis

The cracks in Partnership processes can show quite early on if labor and management partners are not prepared to support joint activities. The Labor-Management Partnership experience at Cook County Health (formerly Cook County Health and Hospitals System) offers an example. Cook County Health, the third-largest public health system in the United States, treating more than 500,000 patients each year, has been struggling for years to provide reasonable access to care for patients. In 2013, labor and management leaders began meeting with a Cornell consultant to develop a partnership process in hopes of improving access to care and improving patient satisfaction. The latter, which was regularly very low, posed a significant problem throughout the delivery system, as hospital reimbursement levels partly depend on patient satisfaction ratings.

For this process, Lazes appointed a consultant who was new to the work of Cornell's Healthcare Transformation Project but quite familiar with Kaiser's Partnership. Cook County union and administrative leaders met with this consultant several times to set initial goals and to agree upon basic ground rules for their work together. They identified improving access to outpatient services, including specialists, and improving outpatient satisfaction scores as the initial areas on which to focus Partnership problem-solving work groups.

Lack of Preparation

Unfortunately, neither labor nor management at Cook County were fully prepared for the Partnership activities. Each group was skeptical about these endeavors, feeling that the other "was not really serious." They did not establish the essential educational activities for frontline staff, supervisors, and senior leaders to prepare for this work, nor did they arrive at a bud get or a clear-cut agreement about the respective roles of management and frontline staff. In addition, the unions involved (SEIU 73, the Doctors Council, and the American Federation of State, County and Municipal Employees local 31) did not create goals for the project that would be to their benefit, as inter-union friction hampered their ability to achieve consensus. Further, neither the unions nor the administration appointed internal consultants to support the new work groups. As a result, the initial work groups floundered due to a lack of training and support, including the fact that they had not been offered enough time to pursue their work. Because of these failures, the Partnership process fizzled out within 18 months.

Given the existing friction between unions and the entrenched hostility between labor and management at Cook County, establishing a good working

Partnership there was destined to be a difficult and arduous process. However, it is regretful that the external consultant assigned to the Partnership, new to Cornell's approach to Partnership implementation and uninterested in receiving guidance about it, failed to fully implement three core practices described in chapter 3. He did not spend enough face time to adequately prepare the constituents for a Partnership process, did not help management work with frontline leaders to identify areas of common interest to which they might be committed, and did not work closely enough with labor and management leaders to guide them in their initial work group process.[271] Finally, he did not emphasize the need for hiring or developing internal consultants, particularly since his available time to follow through on their process was limited. Some of these failures seemed to occur because the consultant appeared to be skeptical from the beginning that the process could succeed in this setting, preferring to focus his time in another hospital system.

The history of this particular failure underscores the necessity of employing all core practices, and especially the importance of patiently educating and cultivating each constituency group during the initial steps of their collaboration. It never pays to initiate problem-solving groups without first preparing leadership and frontline staff for the endeavor. In the end, however, some sites are simply not ready or able to make a joint commitment to the Labor-Management Partnership process, as a result of biased leadership or of a genuine inability to commit adequate resources to it.

Too-Rapid Change Leading to a False Start

Another factor that can contribute to an LMP failing early in the process, even after having established basic goals, ground rules, and work teams, is a too-hasty attempt at change. For example, study teams need to carefully prepare employees whose jobs may be altered through the process before they finalize and attempt to implement their recommendations.

An example of such an omission occurred several years ago at a small hospital in central Harlem, New York, whose Partnership was initiated with the goal of improving overall patient care. Gene McCabe, the CEO of North General Hospital, and Betty Hughley, the vice president of SEIU 1199, were co-leaders able to elicit both labor and management support for a Partnership process at this site. Both were well-liked, their enthusiasm for starting a Labor-Management Partnership process was well received by frontline staff, and their positive and uplifting spirit was contagious in this small community hospital.

Two initial problem-solving groups were established after a half-day meeting held to launch the Partnership process. One work group focused on reducing patient wait times in the outpatient department; a second attempted to reduce turnaround time for laboratory results. These two work groups started immediately brainstorming possible solutions. Frontline staff in the two groups were extremely enthusiastic about the opportunity to make changes that would improve patient care and rapidly developed potential solutions to their assigned problems.

Unfortunately, neither group consulted with those staff whose jobs would need to change if their proposed solutions were implemented. As a result, most frontline workers in the two departments where the problem-solving teams were focused refused to consider their recommendations. Although senior management and union leaders at the hospital felt that Partnership activities would eventually have value for both patients and staff, the false start led to North General Hospital terminating Partnership activities at that point.

Importance of Consulting with Affected Staff

This experience underlines another important practice to keep in mind in partnership work. At Xerox, Study Action Team members constantly interacted with the shop-floor members whose work their recommendations would eventually affect. Work groups who anticipate promoting significant changes in work practices need to introduce their data and reasoning and to obtain feedback from affected staff as their work progresses, rather than presenting the involved staff a fait accompli. This constitutes an important aspect of collaborative leadership: those designated to make significant workplace changes, even if they are managers and frontline staff working in tandem, need to consult with staff who will be affected before recommending significant changes.

Both Partners Need to Participate

Another example of a challenge to establishing an LMP process can be found when only one of the two partners is willing to engage in joint work. This recently occurred at the Cambridge Health Alliance in Cambridge, Massachusetts, a community-based healthcare delivery system just outside of Boston. Two unions representing workers in the Alliance (CIR and the Union of Social Workers, a local union of AFSCME) made frequent attempts over a six-year period to encourage senior management to enter a joint process for improving patient care. The two areas suggested were (1) improving access to behavioral health services and (2) addressing the dilemmas caused by inadequate health insurance reimbursements for patients needing behavioral healthcare.

Although initially seeming receptive to establishing a joint process, the Alliance administration was ultimately unwilling to agree to a joint process. Some psychiatrists and primary care doctors in the administration favored such an endeavor, but their support was superseded by senior management, who preferred to respond to these challenges solely through their own initiatives.[272] Lacking a partner, the unions retreated from their proposal, yet they remain hopeful that they will eventually convince management of the value of working together.[273]

Sabotage by Those Feeling Left Behind by Change

Apart from process failures, or those related to difficulties in gaining the full commitment of management or union leaders, our research and that of others suggests that certain difficulties within organizational cultures are particularly hard to overcome in sustaining Partnership processes.[274] In systems that have developed a "hybrid organization," in which some parts of a large system adopt cooperative work structures, while others continue to work with the traditional top-down arrangement, the asymmetry may breed unhealthy discontent, envy, and competition.

This was the case at the Saturn plant in Spring Hill, Tennessee, described in chapter 3, which was organized on a team-based work system with extensive frontline participation and a nonadversarial labor relations system.[275] Saturn's labor agreement included provisions for multi-skilled, flexible jobs and profit-sharing. Over time, this agreement became increasingly perceived as a threat by the United Auto Workers union's new national leadership, who were unfamiliar with the rationale for the agreement and suspicious of the entire Partnership process.

Simultaneously, new senior General Motors management became hostile to how the Saturn plant was structured, with freedom to design its own cars and access to significant, separate funding from GM.[276] They were concerned that workers and plant managers elsewhere at GM might demand similar labor decision-making authority. Facing financial pressures in early 2000 resulting from the over-capacity of other GM assembly plants and a dip in sales of small cars, senior GM managers reduced production at the Saturn plant, despite its strong market share and strong customer loyalty.[277] They stopped Saturn engineers from updating the car design and forbade them from exploring the manufacture of new Saturn models, such as midsize cars and SUVs. These decisions resulted in a steady decline in production at the plant. In 2010, GM management decided to stop manufacturing Saturn cars.

Thus, late in Saturn's tenure, the national leadership of the UAW and of GM changed. Most of the new leaders had not participated in Saturn's founding, felt uncomfortable with the culture that had been established there, and had more traditional mindsets and biases, which viewed union and management as adversaries.[278] These new leaders actively opposed the Partnership process from the start. Interpersonal conflicts between the local union leadership at Saturn (UAW Local 1853) and national UAW leaders had also developed. As a result, the national union never fought the increasing restrictions on Saturn's production or GM's decision to halt production of the car.

Clashes of Cultures and Regression in Groups

One aspect of these decisions seems rooted in the human tendency to retreat to traditional solutions when conflict arises or when economic pressures move organizations to cut back. However, other forces may also be at work when traditionalists wage war with perceived upstarts. In chapter 5, we illustrate how such a war within an organization can happen: a "fight" regression may occur when a business is challenged economically, beginning with a search for an external or internal scapegoat to blame. Often this may be a subgroup that is already the object of envy or misunderstanding. The regression inflames the emotions of workers who fear for their jobs and leaders who feel pressed to arrive at a solution, which often prevents them from making a focused, unbiased analysis of all contributing factors.

The tendency to isolate and exclude the "new" group is exacerbated when a real pay disparity exists between workers with new, evolving jobs that carry increased responsibility and those remaining in lower paying, more mundane positions without advancement opportunities. This wage and decision-making discrepancy took place in the coal mines of the UK and at Volvo, as discussed in chapter 2.

Anticipating and preparing for this potential clash of cultures in any hybrid system is crucial. Such culture clashes tend to occur when an organization becomes challenged economically, testing its commitment to the new processes; when wage and decision-making differences stir up workers on opposing sides of the pay and advancement differential; or when intraunion difficulties arise in a multiple-union system.[279] The latter has been the case recently at Kaiser, where conflict among its unions may impair their frontline-staff work group process. We discuss this possibility shortly. In such cases, the tendency to find blame in the "newfangled" work system, coupled with momentum to keep the old, more familiar, culture, may override attention to the merits of new process.

Another example of the challenge posed by different, coexisting, work cultures was seen at Rushton Mining Company, a coal mine in Osceola Mills, central Pennsylvania, in the early 1970s. Arnold Miller, then president of the United Mine Workers of America, wondered whether Eric Trist's work with coal miners in England, described in chapter 2, might benefit his members. After securing an agreement with Warren Hicks, Rushton's president, and with the local union membership to establish new work systems that might improve mine safety and overall productivity, Miller oversaw the establishment of several self-managed sections of the mining operation. The remaining sections operated in more traditional ways. These sections of the mine were monitored for a year on safety issues, including reported accidents; on absences; on productivity; and on maintenance costs, as well as on the daily tonnage of mined coal products.[280] If the self-managing production proved helpful, then the entire mine would shift to this production process.

The results of the research, conducted a year after pi lot work groups were established, revealed that the self-managed work groups had fewer safety problems, experienced a significant reduction in lost-time accidents and absenteeism, and achieved slightly greater production numbers than other sections of the mine. Interviews with mine workers in the self-managed work groups revealed that they felt extremely proud of their work, felt recognized for their good ideas by their co-workers, and were "no longer tired after getting home."[281] Despite the positive outcomes, though, union members voted down a proposal in 1974, a year after the implementation of the new work system, to expand self-managing work groups to the entire mine. Many workers feared that expanding the new system would give only the most senior, experienced workers the interesting jobs and increased pay within the new structure.

This fear arose because miners who participated in the initial self-managed work groups had begun to receive pay increases, as many of them were now performing multiple jobs. If other areas of the mine formed self-managing work groups, these miners would have obtained similar increases in pay, but envy of the higher-paid colleagues and overall anxiety about losing out seemed to override this calculation. Further, some foremen described fearing loss of their influence at the mine if the self-managing work groups expanded and hence did not support the process.[282]

These examples suggest that LMP leaders must anticipate organizational regressions that can occur due to members' anxieties about the loss of familiar theories and practices, and about losing power, prestige, or economic benefits in the new system. In the face of such anxieties, constituents may favor the old, even when confronted with data that identify a superior, potentially more remunerative, process.

It is therefore important that Partnership leaders continue to nurture relations with senior union leaders (particularly with the national union president, as in the Saturn example) and with senior management leaders throughout the LMP process (again seen at Saturn). It is wise to ensure that Partnership processes will enable all employees to eventually have the ability to work in new ways and receive similar pay, overall benefits, and decision-making capability—not just those in the initial work groups. Otherwise, resentment is created between those who have garnered the new opportunities and those who have not. One cannot assume that the workforce will automatically understand such future benefits. At Maimonides, employing continual reinforcement about the gains that workers have made within the new systems, and built-in reminders to new managers about their value, have helped to prevent such misreadings. Without a clear strategy to prepare for and address such possibilities, the Labor-Management Process is put at risk.

Responding to Challenges

Even when implementing less radical work systems or quality improvement initiatives, challenges may still threaten their being sustained. At Kaiser, the Los Angeles County Department of Health Services, and Maimonides Medical Center, some frontline staff voiced resentment at not having the opportunity to participate in an Action Team, a particular work group, or a unit-based team. Addressing these concerns immediately resolved the conflict between those inside and those outside the process. Importantly, in the face of such resentment, leaders in these change processes found ways to include frontline staff more widely in their projects. It seems apparent that employees who feel denied opportunities will subvert implementation of the new systems from which they feel excluded.

Besides cultural or economic changes, changes in union and management leaders can greatly affect whether healthcare LMP practices are sustained or eliminated. Again, employee participation activities are time-consuming and require the commitment of both union and management senior leaders to support the process. Although there is no foolproof vaccination against a potential disruption caused by a change in labor or management leaders, a clear social contract between labor and management about the goals, structures, and resources for joint activities can help sustain a healthcare Labor-Management Partnership process through times of stress. At Maimonides Medical Center, the fact that SEIU 1199 had defined from the outset how Partnership activities would achieve union-building outcomes helped to sustain the Partnership even when senior union leadership at the hospital changed. Similarly, when Dr. Mitch Katz, the director who had instituted the Partnership process at LA-DHS, left his position in April 2018, the already-established governance process and funding arrangement sanctioned by the Board of Supervisors of L.A. County[283] to support Partnership activities served to keep their Partnership process alive.

The need to create support for new work systems entails ongoing education of both leaders and frontline staff and requires continuous communication about the results it has achieved. Just as democratic forms of government require constant struggle and revival, so the educational and communicative processes of Partnerships must function throughout their duration. A lapse in these practices risks the entire endeavor.

A final example of a challenge facing a healthcare LMP is now occurring at Kaiser Permanente. The initial labor group involved in creating the LMP, the Coalition of Kaiser Permanente Unions, represented workers from the 22 major local unions. After 21 years of their Partnership process, significant conflicts developed among the participating unions. Ten unions (Hawaii Nurses and Healthcare Professionals, International Brotherhood of Teamsters, International Longshore and Ware house Union, International Union of Operating Engineers, Kaiser Permanente Nurse Anesthetists Association, Oregon Federation of Nurses and Health Professionals (AFT), United Food and Commercial Workers, United Steelworkers, Unite Here, United Nurses Associations of California/Union of Health Care Professionals) decided to leave the coalition in October 2018 to form their own organization, the Alliance of Health Care Unions. This split in the union coalition stemmed not from issues within the Kaiser Partnership process itself but from fights among the unions concerning leadership and decision making within their coalition.

It is not clear to what extent this rift will affect frontline staff participation and the overall Kaiser Labor-Management Partnership process. Frontline staff continue their involvement in the unit-based teams, in which both the Coalition and the Alliance now represent workers.[284] The Kaiser Partnership process needs to anticipate the impact that these new developments may have in their work going forward, and needs to interface with each union group to ensure that neither withdraws from the Partnership.

Here again, founding agreements that have a history of implementation over time may help considerably to sustain their work.

Throughout this book, we have outlined strategies that can overcome resistance to positive organizational disruption. As David Bornstein, in his book *How to Change the World,* states,

> The capacity to cause change grows in an individual over time, as small-scale efforts lead gradually to larger ones. But the process needs a beginning—a story, an example, an early taste of success — something along the way that helps a person form the belief that it is possible to make the world a better place. Those who act on that belief spread it to others. They are highly contagious. Their stories must be told.[285]

Summary

In this chapter, we reviewed research from Scandinavia and from Maimonides Medical Center indicating that staff who participate in workplace activities that increase their conflict-resolving, analytic, and communication skills are more apt to engage in civic involvements outside the job. This is crucial, since widespread civic alienation and disengagement has become quite destructive to American democracy.

We also analyzed the failures of two Labor-Management Partnerships with an eye toward preventing their recurrence in the future. One Partnership did not engage in central core practices, particularly those about preparing both labor and management for their endeavor: educating administrators and union officials about what is possible and helping them to establish workable goals. That Partnership also did not provide adequate assistance to their teams.

In another setting, a very enthusiastic group of staff and administrators quickly launched teams that proposed new ways of organizing work on their units. Without preparing the workers who would have to engage in the new systems, however, the process foundered. When significant changes in work are introduced, it is crucial to have discussed the reasons for and the impact of such alterations with those most affected.

In another situation, despite considerable preparation on the union's part in proposing a Labor-Management Partnership, managers decided to address clinical issues themselves. LMPs are by nature a two-way process. It is to be hoped that the union might be able to convince these administrators in the future of what they have to offer. Unfortunately this will not always be the case.

EPILOGUE

A Call for Collective Action

> You never change things by fighting the existing reality. To change something, build a new model that makes the existing model obsolete.
>
> —*Buckminster Fuller*

As we were writing this book, many doctors and nurses confided in us their absolute distress over the way our healthcare system has shifted in the past 30 years, which they see as depriving them of the opportunity to practice clinical care in a meaningful, professional, and ethical manner. We view them as suffering from a sense of "moral injury." Moral injury constitutes "the damage done to one's conscience or moral compass when ... [a] person perpetrates, witnesses, or fails to prevent acts that transgress one's own moral beliefs, values, or ethical codes of conduct."[286] Originally observed by Jonathan Shay [287] in returning Vietnam War veterans, this phenomenon has been observed by some nurses and doctors within themselves: "The system had bound the physicians so tightly with scheduling control, data and metrics, policies and punishment that they ... could barely breathe. They had almost no control over their patient interactions or their referral options ...

they knew what patients needed but did not have the latitude or the autonomy to get it."[288]

We view our book as *a call for collective action* in the face of such forces, which have created powerful and disruptive incursions into the ability of professional staff to provide patients with the care they need. Patients are forced into the untenable situation of being treated by clinicians who are increasingly hamstrung in their capacities to provide them with personal, professional, and empathic care.

A severe but silent sense of injury dominates our healthcare system as currently constructed. Many administrators fail to recognize this, or when they do, they do not know how to enact meaningful change. Even when observed from a strictly corporate point of view, however, the top-down, siloed methods they use increase costs as well as offering inferior clinical outcomes. "Administrative creep"[289] has overwhelmed most systems, with 10 administrators hired for every physician and an increase in administrative hiring of 3200 percent from 1975 to 2010.[290] Significant costs have accrued from these skyrocketing administrative salaries, as well as from inefficient care processes.[291]

In order to create systems that provide cost-effective, timely, professional, and better-coordinated care, it is essential that healthcare organizations make use of the input of staff at every level. This approach is endorsed by many who study complex organizational structures. *It holds no matter what form of payment is used,* whether a patient has insurance through his or her employer, exercises a public option, or is enrolled in Medicare for All. What is important is to find a payment process in which all Americans have access to healthcare services, healthcare systems are reimbursed for care coordination, and clinicians are not penalized for ethical practices.

Without hearing the voices of their staff, healthcare organizations lack clear-cut methods to fully identify systemic problems in clinical care. In fact, within many hospitals, clinician-employees feel hampered in voicing their concerns from fear of being reprimanded.[292] Fearing censure or dismissals, most practitioners don't speak up. Many use shortcuts such as workarounds, which may be effective in the short run but do nothing to resolve issues in work or care design. (A common example of a workaround is the borrowing of supplies and equipment from other units when they are missing in one's own, or changing procedure coding to obtain payment for extra time spent with a patient.)

When staff, patients, and regulatory organizations are excluded from hospital initiatives for improving access and quality of care, the institution automatically loses essential input. When administrators purchase equipment or software such as electronic medical records systems without consulting with the clinicians who will use them, those clinicians flounder under the weight of the added workload. Electronic medical records, "intended as work-saving tools, have gone in the opposite direction, taking time away from patient care in the name of electronic box-checking."[293] This results in frustration for all.

Maimonides Medical Center and the Los Angeles County Department of Health Services were extremely fortunate to have been graced with visionary leaders who deeply understood the value of collaboration with all of their staff. Senior administrators and union leaders such as Pam Brier and Bruce Richard at Maimonides, and Dr. Mitchell Katz and Patricia Castillo in Los Angeles, were aware of the importance of staff buy-in for the changes they anticipated to be essential for their centers, and they became convinced of the importance of working with their employees to fully identify and correct shortcomings in care.

When healthcare leaders, on the other hand, are cautious, unfamiliar with such methods, biased against labor-management collaboration, hostile toward labor unions, or simply unwilling to share their power, frontline staff and their local unions, such as the AFT's Vermont Federation of Nurses and Health Professionals at the University of Vermont Medical Center, can exert pressure on them to change. While it is extremely difficult to challenge the power of the massive organizations that own chains of hospitals and of large private insurance companies, nonetheless the systems that have succeeded in these endeavors offer proof that collaborative organizational structures benefit hospitals, staff, patients, and the bottom line. These examples need to be trumpeted to all concerned: our political leaders, regulators, and everyone with a stake in the healthcare system. We have shown that healthcare partnerships can benefit patients, staff, and administrators.

A highly structured form of collaboration, LMPs have been shown to successfully tackle systemic problems in healthcare organizations. Several essential practices, described in detail in chapter 3, contribute to their success. These practices include the following:

1. Establishing a social contract between labor and management from the outset that outlines their goals and mutual responsibilities
2. Developing extensive educational activities for frontline staff and senior leaders to familiarize them with the methods and importance of collaborative work
3. Developing internal consultants to oversee and assist the teams charged with identifying and solving problems within the organization
4. Attending to the overall tone and practice of labor relationships within the organization
5. Stressing the importance of documentation and communication of the results of partnership activities

Labor-Management Partnerships have multiple options for approaching organizational change. These include developing teams of frontline staff who identify, analyze, and solve problems with clinical care in their individual units, department-based teams that address issues within an entire department, and Study Action Teams that focus on systemic issues within an entire medical center.

Once teams have been established, it is important for team leaders and internal consultants to be prepared to address the irrational forces that at times can overtake group functioning. Arming teams with knowledge about problem-solving techniques, conflict-resolution strategies, and the basics of workflow analysis will go far to prevent the kinds of irrational forces that can overtake groups when they are unstructured and unprepared for their task.

Nonetheless, it is useful for team leaders to be prepared to work through the impasses that sometimes arise within groups. At times, teams may engage in infighting or in blaming outside forces for their difficulties, may become passive and leave their leader to do all of their work, or may retreat into distracting, gossipy exchanges—all to the detriment of their functioning. We have offered strategies to group leaders and internal consultants that can help them work through these impasses, found in chapter 5.

We have also stressed the importance of understanding and addressing the sensitive issues that arise within groups composed of members from different strata of the power hierarchy and of different ethnicities. In these instances, it is helpful to compose group membership in a way that guarantees that staff at the bottom of the hierarchy are well represented and heard. Group leaders should be coached to make sure that such members feel able to safely contribute their thoughts. Many times, meeting separately with these employees can be helpful in getting them comfortable to share ideas and to speak up in groups with other stakeholders, regardless of who they are.

Once systems have been persuaded to engage in Labor-Management Partnerships and their teams are effectively functioning, other strategies might be enlisted that further enhance workers' autonomy and allow them to contribute to their organizations' bottom lines. In chapters 2 and 7, we outlined strategies employed in Europe and in the United States to encourage staff to develop innovative services, work processes, and technologies that may produce additional income for their hospital system, as well as expand their own job possibilities. Some universities have partnered with these efforts, sharing their own areas of expertise, such as in technology, product development, and marketing. In Europe, unions have actively financed such activities and championed them.

In many hospital settings in the United States, healthcare unions have unfortunately been excluded from exercising such opportunities or have resisted organizing their members to insist on meaningful and clinically ethical work practices. The unions who actively participated in the Allegheny General Hospital, Kaiser Permanente, Los Angeles County Department of Health Services, Maimonides Medical Center, and University of Vermont Medical Center Partnerships, however, created a voice for workers and improved the quality of their work lives. They also increased contact with their members and demonstrated their active value beyond contract negotiations and the handling of grievances. This resulted in increased union membership and increased power for the unions in these healthcare organizations. Many healthcare unions have now developed their own structures to assist in partnership efforts, and it is hoped that these will continue to be used.

Enlisting Healthcare Managers and Administrators into Collaborative Work

We have already mentioned reasons for managers' and administrators' resistance toward partnerships and have discussed the need to exert pressure on them to consider this option. One of the dilemmas with which we have struggled has been to identify alternate approaches to senior managers that might help overcome their resistance to structured collaboration.

Most hospital and healthcare administrators, as well as managers of manufacturing and high-tech companies, lack knowledge about the benefits of structured collaboration as an effective management tool. Clayton Christensen, in his seminal book on what is needed to improve our healthcare systems, *The Innovator's Prescription,* emphasizes that unfortunately "most of the current actors in the health-care industry lack the scale and scope to create a new system architecture."[294]

Healthcare managers have operated, to a large extent, by "keeping the trains running on time," rather than by creating a vision about what troubles their organizations' effective operation and researching methods to redress these. Many managers are low-risk-takers with handsome rewards that they are reluctant to sacrifice. The mean annual compensation for major nonprofit medical center CEOs is now over $3.1 million, 12 times more than pediatricians receive.[295] They tend to justify such salaries by surrounding themselves with the trappings of a power that they are reluctant to share.

It takes vision and courage for them to disrupt the current fee-for-service processes in order to demand that insurers reimburse activities that coordinate care or to insist that insurers alter their electronic medical records requirements to be more clinician-appropriate. As Steve Shortell at the University of California, Berkeley, School of Public Health states, "We are not yet at the tipping point of what is needed to improve healthcare quality or contain costs."[296] Why risk rocking the boat with a new approach when healthcare administrators do not yet face the pressure that will force them to make systemic changes?

It is therefore imperative for organizations such America's Essential Hospitals, the Association of

American Medical Colleges, the American Public Health Association, the American Management Association, and the Labor and Employment Relations Association to educate their constituents about the urgent need for systemic change. These organizations have an obligation to educate themselves and their constituents about the data on successful organizational change methods.

Over the long term, nursing, medical, public health, and business schools should fulfill this obligation by including courses in organizational change, in methods to create new work systems, and in approaches to collaboration with frontline staff. This will help the next generation of healthcare leaders to become more open to and knowledgeable about such approaches to systemic change. Some healthcare unions, such as the Committee of Interns and Residents, the Doctors Council, and the American Federation of Teachers' Nurses and Health Professionals division, are already fulfilling this obligation by requiring their leaders to become educated about these methods.

In the near term, conferences and strategically placed articles and books, such as ours, can be used to encourage healthcare administrators to learn from their colleagues—Mitch Katz, Pam Brier, and others—about practical ways to restructure their operations. We have written in chapter 5 about the reasons why groups tend to hold negative mindsets toward "the other," "the outsider." Such prejudices can powerfully influence leaders against collaboration.

These stances might be affected, however, by their hearing firsthand from peers about actual, positive experiences and their beneficial results.

Apart from emphasizing the intrinsic benefits to healthcare organizations of working collaboratively with their frontline staff, we hope that public health educators will also stress the benefit of such work to their communities. In chapter 8, we reviewed several studies documenting that after participating in frontline staff decision-making activities, employees were much more likely to become actively engaged in civic projects outside of work. This is a highly desirable benefit, as it can strengthen our democratic institutions, which are currently in peril.

In the end, however, the American healthcare "system" is entangled by corporate greed. Pharmaceutical companies feel entitled to jack up prices for medications that are essential to patient care, even when they have been previously available at low cost. Private insurers regard their primary responsibility as meeting their shareholders' needs and as accruing their own profits, rather than as providing a service to their enrolled patients. According to a review of Elizabeth Rosenthal's book *An American Sickness,* "Even nonprofit Medicare and Medicaid now contract out services to some ... [private insurers whose] many tangled plans and subplans have providers bouncing on and off their rosters at warp speed, destroying continuity of care.... Likewise, medications flit on and off approved drug lists, their presence or absence depending on continual negotiations between insurer and manufacturer."[297] As for "nonprofit" hospitals, they often funnel their gains into large executive salaries and new wings or buildings instead of staff salaries and patient care.

It will require *collective action* on the part of healthcare practitioners and patients to insist on disentangling the tentacles of these highly intertwined systems. Rather than giving in to misery or simply leaving the field, these groups must learn that it is up to them to demand change.

We offer in this book a blueprint for one way of reversing the trends of the last 30 years that have strangled our patient care systems. Hopefully, *collective action by those with a stake in actually treating patients (rather than simply enriching themselves), in synchrony with political change,* can help to resurrect a viable American healthcare system.

It is likely that a single-payer coverage system with secondary supplementation for copayments, added drug coverage, and comprehensive behavioral health benefits will create a situation in which everyone will be insured. In this way, coverage will no longer be subject to the Byzantine sign-up conditions and high deductibles of the Obamacare plan and will not be held hostage by for-profit companies. It should also be easier to negotiate costs and conditions, given enough pressure from all stakeholders, with a single entity, as opposed to with multiple players. We await the tipping point at which this will become possible. We hope, given the chaos surrounding patients' coverage throughout the COVID-19 epidemic, that the tipping point may have arrived.

We give the last word to Eleanor Roosevelt:

> Where, after all, do universal human rights begin? In small places close to home—so close and so small they cannot be seen on any maps of the world. Yet they are the world of the individual person; the neighborhood he lives in; the school or college he attends; the factory, farm, or office where he works. Unless these rights have meaning there, they have little meaning anywhere. Without concerned citizen action to uphold them close to home, we shall look in vain for progress in the larger world.[298]

Notes

[1] Dolan, T. (2008) "Newark and Its Gateway Complex, Part 3: A Weakened City." *Newark Metro, Rutgers Online.* http://www.newarkmetro.rutgers.edu/reports/display.php?id=17&page=3; accessed May 25, 2019.

[2] Abrams, M.K. (2014) "Medical Homes: An Evolving Model of Primary Care." *To the Point,* Commonwealth Fund. February 25.

[3] Fisher, R.L. (2020) "A Primary Care Physician at His Peak Is Forced into Early Retirement." *MedPage Today.* January 6, p.2.

[4] LeBlanc, S. (2020) "Baker's State of the Commonwealth Address Goals: Climate, Transportation, Health Care." *Berkshire Eagle.* January 21.

[5] Ofri, D. (2019) "The Business of Health Care Depends on Exploiting Doctors and Nurses." *New York Times.* June 8.

[6] Brown, T., and S. Bergman. (2020) "Our Health Record Mess." *New York Times.* January 1, p. A19.

[7] Conversation with Denise Duncan, president of United Nurses Associations of California, February 25, 2020.

[8] Abelson, R., and M.S. Sanger-Katz. (2019) "Medicare for All Would Abolish Private Insurance. 'There's No Precedent in American History.'" *New York Times.* March 23, p. A1.

[9] Tucker, A.T., S.J. Singer, J.E. Hayes, and A. Falwell. (2008) "Front-Line Staff Perspectives on Opportunities for Improving the Safety and Efficiency of Hospital Work." *Health Services Research* 43, no.5, part 2 (October), p.1826.

[10] In countries such as Sweden, Norway, and Germany, there exists national legislation to give workers the right to participate in workplace decisions.

[11] Elden, M., and M. Levin. (1991) "Cogenerative Learning: Bringing Participation into Action Research." In *Participatory Action Research,* edited by W.F. Whyte. Newbury Park, CA: Sage Publications, pp.127–43.

[12] U.S. Bureau of Labor Statistics, Economic News Release; figures for 2017.

[13] Ibid.

[14] Baily, M.N., and R.Z. Lawrence. (2004) "What Happened to the Great U.S. Job Machine? The Role of Trade and Electronic Offshoring." Washington, DC. *Brookings Papers on Economic Activity* 2, pp.211–84.

[15] Ibid.

[16] Ibid.

[17] The American Federation of Teachers/Nurses and Health Professionals, the Committee of Interns and Residents, Doctors Council, and Service Employees International Union.

[18] Lazes, P., S. Gordon, and S. Samy. (2012) "Excluded Actors in Patient Safety." In *First Do Less Harm: Confronting the Inconvenient Problems of Patient Safety,* edited by R. Koppel and S. Gordon. Ithaca, NY: ILR Press/Cornell University Press, pp.93–122.

[19] Ofri (2019) "The Business of Health Care Depends on Exploiting Doctors and Nurses."

[20] Kania, J., and M. Kramer. (2011) "Collective Impact." *Stanford Social Innovation Review,* Winter, pp.20–29.

[21] Ibid.

[22] Interview with William Quintana, October 12, 2013.

[23] Meaningful work is considered work that is challenging, where one gets feedback in a timely manner. (Hackman, J.R., and G.R. Oldham. 1980 *Work Redesign.* Reading, MA: Addison-Wesley).

[24] Unions such as Amalgamated Clothing and Textile Workers and the United Steelworkers had similar points of view.

[25] Reuther, W. (1941) *500 Planes a Day.* Pamphlet. American Council on Public Affairs, 1941.

[26] Green house, S. (2019) *Beaten Down, Worked Up: The Past, Pre sent, and Future of American Labor.* New York: Alfred A. Knopf, pp.96–97.

[27] Herzberg, F. (1968) "One More Time: How Do You Motivate Employees?" *Harvard Business Review,* pp.46–57.

[28] U.S. Senate Subcommittee on Employment, Manpower, and Poverty, July 25, 1972.

[29] Scheiber, N. (2019) "Workers Chase Spoils of Boom on Picket Lines." *New York Times.* October 20, p.20.

[30] Guest, R.H. (1979) "Quality of Work Life—Learning from Tarrytown." *Harvard Business Review,* sec. 57 (July), pp.15–28.

[31] Ibid.

[32] Ibid.

[33] Hevesi, D. (2007) "Irving Bluestone, 90, Top U.A.W. Negotiator, Dies." *New York Times.* November 21.

[34] Guest, R.H. (1979) "Quality of Work Life—Learning from Tarrytown," p.9.

[35] Ibid., p.9.

[36] Ibid., p.11.

[37] Ibid., p.20.

[38] Greenberg, P.D., and E.M. Glaser. (1980) "Some Issues in Joint Union-Management Quality of Worklife Improvement Efforts." *Psyc-CRITIQUES* 25, no.12 (May), pp.1–95.

[39] Walton, R.E. (1973) "Quality of Working Life: What Is It?" *Sloan Management Review* 15, no.1, pp.11–21.

[40] Ibid.

[41] McLeod, A.D., P. Lillrank, and N. Kano. (1991) "Continuous Improvement: Quality Control Circles in Japanese Industry." *Journal of Asian Studies* 50, no.2, p.416.

[42] QWL teams were not to work on labor contract issues.

[43] Conversation with William Quintana, November 11, 2012.

[44] In fact, their initial consultant, Sid Rubinstein, was trained on the approach of quality control circles and provided the consulting to the Tarrytown GM plant.

[45] Hayward, S.G., B.C. Dale, and V.C.M. Frazer. (1985) "Quality Circle Failure and How to Avoid It." *European Management Journal* 3, no.2, pp.103–11.

[46] Elden, M., and M. Levin. (1991) "Cogenerative Learning."

[47] A sidebar agreement is an agreement between labor and management that becomes part of their labor agreement as an amendment.

[48] Although a job might change, no employee would be laid off as a result of Labor-Management Partnership activities.

[49] In 1997, Kaiser Permanente established a similar worker involvement process that focused on unit-based teams similar to the quality control circles of GM's Tarrytown assembly plant.

[50] Lazes, P., and A. Costanza. (1984) "Xerox Cuts Costs Without Layoffs Through Union-Management Collaboration." U.S. Department of Labor—Bureau of Labor-Management Relations and Cooperative Programs. July, pp.1–7.

[51] Ibid.

[52] Klingel, S., and A. Martin. (1988) *A Fighting Chance: New Strategies to Save Jobs and Reduce Costs.* Ithaca, NY: ILR Press/Cornell University Press.

[53] Lazes, P., and J. Savage. (2000) "Embracing the Future: Union Strategies for the 21st

Century." *Journal for Quality and Participation* 23, no.4 (Fall), pp.18–23.

[54] Reid, R., K. Coleman, E. Johnson, P. Fishman et al. (2010) "The Group Health Medical Home at Year Two: Cost Savings, Higher Patient Satisfaction, and Less Burnout for Providers." *Health Affairs* 29, no.5 (May), pp.835–43.

[55] Ibid., p.841.

[56] Christensen, C.M., J.H. Grossman, and J. Hwang. (2009) *The Innovator's Prescription: A Disruptive Solution for Health Care.* New York: McGraw Hill.

[57] Klingel, S., and A. Martin (1988) *A Fighting Chance.*

[58] Lazes was the consultant for Xerox and ACTWU from 1980 to 1987 and suggested the approach of the SAT process as a method to reduce manufacturing costs.

[59] Maimonides Medical Center. (2007) "Creating Competitive Advantage in a Changing Health Care Environment through Worker Participation: Strategic Alliance Report 2007." Brooklyn, NY: Maimonides Medical Center, p.6.

[60] Christensen, C.M., J.H. Grossman, and J. Hwang. (2009) *The Innovator's Prescription.*

[61] Ibid.

[62] Rae-Dupree, J. (2009) "Disruptive Innovation, Applied to Health Care." *New York Times.* February 1.

[63] Emery, F.E., and E. Thorsrud. (1969) *Form and Content in Industrial Democracy.* London, UK: Tavistock Institute, p.88.

[64] Schiller, B. (1977) "Industrial Democracy in Scandinavia." *Annals of the American Academy of Political and Social Science,* no.431 (May), pp.63–73.

[65] Ibid.

[66] Ibid.

[67] Emery, F.E., and E. Thorsrud. (1969) *Form and Content in Industrial Democracy.*

[68] Ibid., p.188.

[69] Schiller, B. (1977) "Industrial Democracy in Scandinavia," p.69.

[70] Trahair, R. (2015) *Behavior, Technology, and Organizational Development: Eric Trist and the Tavistock Institute.* New Brunswick, NJ: Transaction Publishers.

[71] Trist, E. (1981) *The Evolution of Socio-technical Systems: A Conceptual Framework and an Action Research Program.* Toronto, Canada: Ontario Quality of Working Life Centre.

[72] The Tavistock Institute was established after World War II to determine how to improve the effectiveness of organizations and to understand some of the psychodynamic factors, both in groups and individually, that contribute or weaken these opportunities.

[73] Trahair, R. (2015) *Behavior, Technology, and Organizational Development,* p.143.

[74] Trist and Emery ended up documenting, through numerous papers and several books, how organizations use socio-technical systems as a means for creating more productive work systems and more meaningful work for workers.

[75] Trahair, R. (2015) *Behavior, Technology, and Organizational Development,* p.143.

[76] Sandberg, A. (1994) "Volvoism at the End of the Road? Does the Closing-Down of Volvo's Uddevalla Plant Mean the End of Human-Centered Alternative to a Toyotism?" *The Swedish Center for Working Life.*

[77] These were human resources approaches to help deal with morale issues. Herzberg, Hulin, and Blood were key scholars who identified the importance of job enlargement and enrichment.

[78] Sandberg, A. (1994) "Volvoism at the End of the Road?"

[79] Taylor, L.K. (1973) "Worker Participation in Sweden." *Industrial and Commercial Training* 5, no.1 (January).

[80] Sandberg, A. (1994) "Volvoism at the End of the Road?"

[81] Ibid.

[82] Ibid.

[83] Doing what is needed to get the work done by disregarding current work policies.

[84] Conversation with Kjeld Lisby, November 4, 2015.

[85] More common have been industrial incubators that are used to help innovate and bring new products to market quickly.

[86] Interview with Kristine Rasmussen, November 2, 2015.

[87] Interview with Jasper Bredmose Simasen, November 4, 2015.

[88] Interview with Kjeld Lisby, November 4, 2015.

[89] Anderson, I. (1996) "Ethics and Health Research in Aboriginal Communities." In *Ethical Intersections: Health Research, Methods and Researcher Responsibility,* edited by Jeanne Daly. Sydney, Australia: Allen & Unwin Press, pp.513–65.

[90] Baum, F., C. MacDougall, and D. Smith. (2006) "Participatory Action Research." *Journal of Epidemiology and Community Health* 60, no.10 (Oct.), pp.854–57.

[91] Ibid., p.856.

[92] Ibid., p.857.

[93] Weisbord, M. (2004) *Productive Workplaces Revisited: Dignity, Meaning, and Community in the 21st Century.* San Francisco: Jossey-Bass.

[94] Putnam, R.D., and L.M. Feldstein. (2003) *Better Together: Restoring the American Community.* New York: Simon & Schuster.

[95] Maimonides Medical Center (2007) "Creating Competitive Advantage in a Changing Health Care Environment through Worker Participation."

[96] Lazes was the director of the Healthcare Transformation Project at Cornell's ILR School from 2007 to 2016.

[97] Interview, W. Edwards Deming and Bill Scherkenbach, February 15, 1984: "The Leadership We Need in Our Organizations."

[98] Collaborative leadership is a style of organizational management that fosters the roles of labor and management as co-leaders who encourage frontline staff to share their knowledge and expertise about problems in their institution. Collaborative leaders enable

staff to identify and solve problems that they experience firsthand and to implement their solutions. Such an approach encourages staff to eventually become leaders in their organization.

[99] Richard, B. (2015) *The Other New York: A Story About Human Transformation.* Kingston, NY: Bruce Richard.

[100] Rubinstein, S., and T. Kochan. (2001) *Learning from Saturn: Possibilities for Corporate Governance and Employee Relations.* Ithaca, NY: ILR Press/Cornell University Press, p.19.

[101] New York State Nurses Association (NYSNA) joined the partnership soon after it officially was started by Pam Brier and John Reid.

[102] Focus group of co-chairs conducted on November 3, 2007.

[103] Maimonides Medical Center. (2007) "Creating Competitive Advantage in a Changing Health Care Environment through Worker Participation."

[104] The unions at Maimonides included SEIU 1199, representing workers other than nurses; the New York State Nurses Association, representing nurses; and the Committee of Interns and Residents, representing interns and residents.

[105] Rudden, M.G., P. Lazes, and J. Newman. (2013) "The Impact of Social Hierarchies on Efforts at Organizational Change: Comparing Two Approaches from the Tavistock Institute for Human Relations." *International Journal of Applied Psychoanalytic Studies* 10, no.3, pp.267–84.

[106] The Labor-Management Project was created by the League of Voluntary Hospitals and Homes of New York and SEIU 1199 in 1999 to assist League hospitals and nursing homes to develop Labor-Management Partnership activities.

[107] Kania, J., and M. Kramer. (2013) "Embracing Emergence: How Collective Impact Addresses Complexity." *Stanford Social Innovation Review.* January 21, pp.1–7.

[108] Interview with Diane Factor, September 15, 2016.

[109] I, along with other colleagues from the Healthcare Transformation Project of Cornell's ILR School, provided research assistance to Maimonides' Labor-Management Partnership Process.

[110] Interview with Susan Goldberg, October 15, 2015.

[111] Interview with a senior executive of LA-DHS, May 12, 2014.

[112] Brown, T. (2018) "Fixing American's Health Care System." *American Journal of Nursing* 118, no.11 (November), p.62.

[113] Conversation with Gilda Valdez, July 14, 2015.

[114] The Medicaid waiver provided additional funds to Los Angeles County for upward of 250,000 uninsured patients.

[115] Abrams, M.K. (2014) "Medical Homes: An Evolving Model of Primary Care."

[116] Improving the patient experience focuses primarily on patient satisfaction scores—which measure how satisfied patients are receiving care.

[117] Gesulga, J., A. Berjame, K.S. Moquiala, and A. Galido. (2017) "Barriers to Electronic Health Record System Implementation and Information System Resources: A Structured Review." *Procedia Computer Science* 124 (2017), pp.544–51.

[118] Interview with Patricia Castillo, director of health services, SEIU Local 721, May 11, 2015.

[119] Ibid.

[120] Interview with Nicole Moore, director of CITs at LA-DHS, October 15, 2016.

[121] Ibid.

[122] California's Section 1115 Medicaid Waiver Public Hospital Redesign and Incentives in the Medi-Cal (PRIME) program requires the County of Los Angeles to meet or exceed 74 health measures covering a range of activities such as cancer screening and chronic disease management. In 2018, LA-DHS earned 99 percent of available incentive funding available through the PRIME program, amounting to over $222 million. Projects initiated by individual CITs and spread to the rest of the MLK facility have shown sustained improvement, with demonstrated gains in each year of the PRIME program.

[123] Material obtained from the Los Angeles County Productivity and Quality Commission—Certificate of Recognition, October 16, 2019.

[124] Conference call with Dr. David Campa, March 13, 2019.

[125] Ibid.

[126] The King Outpatient Center's patient satisfaction scores from July 2018 to July 2019.

[127] LA-DHS funds paid for training staff for new jobs, for 15 internal consultants (Healthcare Transformation Advocates), and for frontline staff to attend educational workshops and to

become members of work groups or CITs. SEIU Local 721 and SEIU International paid for Lazes, the external consultant.

[128] Interview with Wilson Mendez, July 14, 2015.

[129] McCarthy, D., and K. Mueller. (2008) "The New York City Health and Hospitals Corporation: Transforming a Public Safety Net Delivery System to Achieve Higher Performance." Commonwealth Fund. October.

[130] Lazes, P., L. Katz, and M. Figueroa. (2012) *How Labor-Management Partnerships Improve Patient Care, Cost Control, and Labor Relations.* Washington, DC: American Rights at Work, p.7.

[131] Kania, J., and M. Kramer. (2013) "Embracing Emergence."

[132] Kochan, T.A., A.E. Eaton, R.B. McKersie, and P.S. Adler. (2009) *Healing Together: The Labor-Management Partnership at Kaiser Permanente.* Ithaca, NY: ILR Press/Cornell University Press.

[133] Conversation with Marie-Cecile Charlier, October 19, 2007.

[134] Ibid.

[135] SEIU 1199 and the League of Voluntary Hospitals and Homes of New York set aside funds to provide training and consulting to

hospitals and nursing homes to create Labor-Management Partnerships for members of the League.

[136] As result of Marie-Cecile Charlier's leadership in the lab, she become a shop steward for 1199 and then was appointed to the position of a Developer (e.g., internal consultant) to help support various partnership initiatives.

[137] MedPAC Commission. (2008) *Engaging Front Line Staff in Changes to Improve Patient Safety and Quality of Care—Lessons from the Field—Maimonides Medical Center.* Presentation to MedPAC Commissioners. Washington, DC, October 31.

[138] Interview with Louise Valero, October 6, 2006.

[139] The resource group at Maimonides Medical Center included four full-time internal consultants/Developers as well as union staff and management involved in quality improvement initiatives and Maimonides' chief learning officer.

[140] Interview with Pam Brier. January 12, 2016.

[141] MedPAC Commission (2008) *Engaging Front Line Staff in Changes to Improve Patient Safety and Quality of Care.*

[142] Klingel, S., and A. Martin. (1988) *A Fighting Chance.*

[143] System changes involve multiple groups in an organization that are interrelated.

[144] Xerox established their Labor-Management Partnership process in 1980.

[145] Lazes, P., and A. Costanza. (1984) "Xerox Cuts Costs Without Layoffs Through Union-Management Collaboration."

[146] Klingel, S., and A. Martin (1988) *A Fighting Chance,* p.15.

[147] Lazes, P., and A. Costanza. (1984) "Xerox Cuts Costs Without Layoffs Through Union-Management Collaboration."

[148] Ibid., p.4.

[149] Ibid.

[150] Conversation with Bill Asher, July 17, 1984.

[151] Lazes, P., and A. Costanza. (1984) "Xerox Cuts Costs without Layoffs through Labor-Management Collaboration."

[152] Ibid.

[153] Klingel, S., and A. Martin. (1988) *A Fighting Chance.*

[154] Maimonides Medical Center (2007) "Creating Competitive Advantage in a Changing Health Care Environment through Worker Participation."

[155] Bluestone, I. (1976) "A Changing View of Union-Management Relations." *Vital Speeches.* December 11.

[156] Rae-Dupree, J. (2009) "Disruptive Innovation, Applied to Health Care," p. B3.

[157] Emery, F., and E. Thorsrud. (1976) *Democracy at Work: The Report of the Norwegian Industrial Democracy Program.* Leiden, the Netherlands: H.E. Stenfert Kroese.

[158] Rudden, M., P. Lazes, and J. Neumann (2013). "The Impact of Social Hierarchies on Efforts at Organizational Change."

[159] Organizational consultants trained at the Tavistock Institute (reflected in papers edited by Trist and Murray [1990]), at the A.K. Rice Institute (see Colman, A., and M. Geller, eds.[1985] *Group Relations Reader 2.* A.K. Rice Institute) and psychoanalysts influenced by them (Kernberg, O.[1998]) all discuss these basic principles.

[160] Eisold, K., (2010). *What You Don't Know You Know: Our Hidden Motives in Life, Business, and Everything Else.* New York: Other Press.

[161] Kaës, R. (2007) *Linking, Alliances, and Shared Space: Groups and the Psychoanalyst.* New York: International Psychoanalytical Association.

[162] Hopper, E. (2003) "The Fourth Basic Assumption: Incohesion: Aggregation/Massification or (ba) I:A/M." In *Traumatic Experience in the Unconscious Life of Groups,* edited by E. Hopper. London, UK: Jessica Kingsley Publishers, pp.91–107.

[163] Shapiro, R. (1991) "Psychoanalytic Theory of Groups and Organizations."*Journal of the American Psychoanalytic Association* 39, pp.759–82.

[164] Rudden, M., S. Twemlow, and S. Ackerman. (2008) "Leadership and Regressive Group Processes: A Pi lot Study." *International Journal of Psychoanalysis* 89: 993–1010.

[165] Gustafson, J., and L. Cooper. (1985) "Collaboration in Small Groups: Theory and Technique for the Study of Small Group Processes." In Colman, A., and M. Geller, eds. *Group Relations Reader 2,* pp.139–50.

[166] Rudden, M., S. Twemlow, and S. Ackerman. (2008) "Leadership and Regressive Group Processes: A Pi lot Study."

[167] McClelland, D.C. (1985) *Human Motivation.* Glenview, IL: Scott, Foresman.

[168] Hersey, P., and K. Blanchard. (1996) *Management of Organizational Behavior: Utilizing Human Resources.* Englewood Cliffs, NJ: Prentice Hall.

[169] Shapiro, R. (1991) "Psychoanalytic Theory of Groups and Organizations."

[170] Twemlow, S., and F. Sacco. (2013) "How and Why Does Bystanding Have Such a Startling Impact on the Architecture of School Bullying and Violence?" *International Journal of Applied Psychoanalytic Studies* 10, no.3, pp.289–306.

[171] Rudden, M., S. Twemlow, and S. Ackerman. (2008) "Leadership and Regressive Group Processes: A Pi lot Study."

[172] Ibid., 1005.

[173] Eckert, R., M. West, D. Altman, K. Steward, and B. Pasmore. (2014) "Delivering a Collective Leadership Strategy for Health Care." The King's Fund, Center for Creative Leadership, p.1.

[174] Rudden, M., P. Lazes, and J. Neumann. (2013) "The Impact of Social Hierarchies on Efforts at Organizational Change," p.280.

[175] Ibid.

[176] Green house, S. (2019) *Beaten Down, Worked Up.*

[177] Bognar, S., and J. Reichert. (2019) "'American Factory': When a Chinese Company Takes Over an Ohio Factory." Washington, DC: High Ground Productions and Netflix. NPR. org, August 21, 2019. Also: Parnass, L. (2018)

"BMC Nurses Call New Strike, Prompting Hospital to Pull 'Generous' Offer." *Berkshire Eagle,* Pittsfield, Massachusetts. June 5, p.24.

[178] Appelbaum, E., and L. Hunter. (2004) "Union Participation in Strategic Decisions of Corporations." In *Emerging Labor Market Institutions for the Twenty-First Century,* by R.B. Freeman, J. Hersch, and L. Michel. Chicago: University of Chicago Press.

[179] U.S. Bureau of Labor Statistics. *Union Members 2017—Union Member Summary.* January 19, 2018.

[180] Green house, S. (2019) *Beaten Down, Worked Up,* p.217.

[181] *Janus v. AFSCME* Supreme Court decision, June 27, 2018. This decision required employees to decide whether or not to pay union dues, although the union was still responsible for representing them if they had a grievance. These employees also received any increase in pay that was negotiated by the union.

[182] Rolf, D. (2018) *A Roadmap to Rebuilding Worker Power.* New York: Century Foundation, p.4.

[183] Conversation with Kris Rondeau, president of Union Share, June 13, 2018.

[184] Many countries in Europe have laws requiring companies over a certain size to have worker representatives on their board of directors or work council.

[185] Rolf, D. (2018) *A Roadmap to Rebuilding Worker Power,* p.88.

[186] Freeman, R., and J. Rogers. (1999) *What Workers Want.* Ithaca, NY: Cornell University Press.

[187] Lazes, P., L. Katz, and M. Figueroa. (2012) *How Labor-Management Partnerships Improve Patient Care, Cost Control, and Labor Relations.*

[188] U.S. Bureau of Labor Statistics. (2018) *Union Members 2017—Union Member Summary.* January 19.

[189] https://wikipedia.org/wiki/Sidney_Hillman.

[190] Schwartz, R. (2006) *The Legal Rights of Union Stewards,* 4th ed. Chicago: Labor Notes.

[191] Tony Kallevig, presentation in Melbourne, Australia, May 26, 2016.

[192] Conference call with Deb Snell, president of the Vermont Federation of Nurses and Health Professionals, June 19, 2019.

[193] Contract language for Unit Collaborative process at University of Vermont Medical Center.

[194] Conversation with Mike Bennet, August 15, 2016.

[195] A recent confrontation between labor and management leaders in Los Angeles took place in fall 2016. The union (SEIU 721) and management couldn't reach an agreement on wage increases for several categories of workers, although the Labor-Management Partnership was quite significant between these parties. This impasse almost resulted in a major strike.

[196] Kallevig, T. (2016) Presentation in Melbourne, Australia, May 26, 2016.

[197] Nembhard, I.M., I.A. Alexander, T.J. Hoff, and R. Ramanujam. (2009) "Why Does the Quality of Health Care Continue to Lag? Insights from Management Research." *Academy of Management Perspectives* (February), pp.24–42.

[198] Walston, S.L., P. Lazes, and P.G. Sullivan. (2004) "Improving Hospital Restructuring: Lessons Learned." *Health Care Management Review* 29, no.4, pp.1–12.

[199] Huzzard, T.D. Gregory, and R. Scott, eds. (2004) *Strategic Unionism and*

Partnership—Boxing or Dancing? New York: Palgrave Macmillan.

[200] Interview with Eric Scherzer, executive director, Committee of Interns and Residents, January 15, 2018.

[201] Lazes, P., N. Gregg, and D. Gamble. (2013) *Worker Voice, Unions and Economic Development.* New York: Ford Foundation.

[202] Conversation with Patricia Castillo, December 1, 2016.

[203] A work-around is a bypass of a recognized problem or limitation in a system.

[204] Nurse practitioners and midwives eventually became members of SEIU 1199 as a result of the partnership process.

[205] Maimonides Medical Center. (2007) "Creating Competitive Advantage in a Changing Health Care Environment through Worker Participation," p.17.

[206] Ibid.

[207] Appelbaum, E., and L. Hunter. (2004) "Union Participation in Strategic Decisions of Corporations."

[208] For contract negotiations, the common approach involves analyzing the strengths and weaknesses of the organization with which

the union is negotiating, in order to prepare demands and to strategize ways to pressure an organization to accept them. When preparing an organizing campaign, research activities attempt to identify ways to persuade frontline staff to join the union.

[209] Lazes, P., and J. Savage. (2000) "Embracing the Future," p.20.

[210] Conversation with Patricia Castillo, December 1, 2016.

[211] The Committee of Interns and Residents (CIR) is the largest house staff union in the United States, representing close to 14,000 interns, residents, and fellows in California, Florida, Massachusetts, New Jersey, New York, New Mexico, and Washington, DC.

[212] The Doctors Council, an affiliate of Service Employees International Union, represents attending doctors in institutions in New York, New Jersey, Illinois, and Pennsylvania.

[213] SEIU Healthcare Pennsylvania is the state's largest and fastest-growing union of nurses and healthcare workers, uniting nearly 45,000 nurses, professional and technical employees, direct care workers, and service employees in hospitals, skilled nursing facilities, home-and community-based services, and state facilities across the Commonwealth.

[214] Conversation with Eric Scherzer, former executive director, CIR, May 17, 2017.

[215] The Coalition of Unions of Kaiser Permanente was the initial group representing all of the unions participating in Partnership activities. The California Nurses Association and the National Union of Healthcare Workers did not participate in the Kaiser Partnership at any time. In 2018, several major unions left the Coalition of Unions and formed their own organization association—the Alliance of Health Care Unions. More details about this new organization are in chapter 8.

[216] Conversation with Josh Rutkoff, former area director, Coalition of Kaiser Permanente Unions, March 20, 2019.

[217] Most unions in the United States are referred to as international unions, although this really means they operate for the most part as national organizations.

[218] Ovretveit, J., P. Bate, P. Cleary et al. (2002) "Quality Collaboratives: Lessons from Research." *Quality and Safety in Health Care* 11, no.4, pp.345–51.

[219] I (Lazes) was the director of Cornell's Healthcare Transformation Project.

[220] Conversation with Bruce Richard, January 17, 2017.

[221] Edmondson, A.C. (2019) *The Fearless Organization: Creating Psychological Safety in the Workplace for Learning, Innovation, and Growth.* Hoboken, NJ: John Wiley and Sons, Inc.

[222] Los Angeles County Health Agency Just Culture Policy. (2017) August 14.

[223] Conversation with Fran Todd, nurse practitioner at LA-DHS, October 16, 2016.

[224] Ibid.

[225] Rolf, D. (2018) *A Roadmap to Rebuilding Worker Power.*

[226] U.S. Senate Subcommittee on Employment, Manpower, and Poverty. July 25, 1972, CB 19-141.

[227] Reid, T.R. (2009) *The Healing of America: A Global Quest for Better, Cheaper, and Fairer Health Care.* New York: Penguin Press.

[228] Christensen, C.M., J.H. Grossman, and J. Hwang. (2009) *The Innovator's Prescription.*

[229] Weisbord, M. (2004) *Productive Workplaces Revisited.*

[230] Conversation with Carmen Rojas, CEO and co-founder of the Worker Lab, August 26, 2019.

[231] Interview with David Rolf, December 14, 2017.

[232] Barton, Laura. (2012) "Hand Sanitizers: Saved by the Gel?" *The Guardian.* May 13.

[233] Smith, A. (2014) "The Lucas Plan: What Can It Tell Us About Democratizing Technology Today?" *The Guardian.* January 22.

[234] Cooley, M. (1980) *Architect or Bee? The Human/Technology Relationship.* Boston. South End Press.

[235] Ibid.

[236] Lazes, P. (1985) "Innovative Approaches to Saving and Creating Jobs." *National Productivity Review.* Spring, pp.146–54.

[237] Transformative changes are radical interventions that result in making prior processes obsolete.

[238] Interview with Stu Winby, October 16, 2017.

[239] Weisbord, M. (2004) *Productive Workplaces Revisited.*

[240] Worley, C.G., S.A. Mohrman, and J.A. Nevitt. (2011) "Large Group Interventions: An Empirical Field Study of Their Composition, Process, and Outcomes." *Journal of Applied Behavioral Science* 47, no.4, pp.404–31.

[241] Kaplan, S. (2012) *Leapfrogging: Harness the Power of Surprise for Business Breakthroughs.* San Francisco: Berrett-Koehler Publishers.

[242] Improving the patient experience is based on direct patient feedback and patient satisfaction scores.

[243] An iterative process is an approach to achieve substantial changes based on systematic, repetitive activities done until a desired outcome is achieved.

[244] One of the important large system approaches is described in Weisbord, M., and S. Janoff (2000), *Future Search: An Action Guide to Finding Common Ground in Organizations and Communities.* San Francisco: Berrett-Koehler Publishers.

[245] Worley, C.G., S.A. Mohrman, and J.A. Nevitt. (2011) "Large Group Interventions," p.421.

[246] Ibid.

[247] Winby, S., and C.G. Worley. (2014) "Management Processes for Agility, Speed, and Innovation." *Organizational Dynamics* 43, no.3, pp.225–34.

[248] Interview with Terry Carroll, Fairview Health Services, September 16, 2016.

[249] Worley, C.G., S.A. Mohrman, and J.A. Nevitt. (2011) "Large Group Interventions," p.426.

[250] Winby, S. (2017) *Sociotechnical Digital Design.* USC Marshall Center for Effective Organizations. April, pp.1–30.

[251] Lazes, P., L.H. Kaplan, and K.A. Gordon. (1987) *The Handbook of Health Education,* 2nd ed. Rockville, MD: Aspen Publishers.

[252] Gruessner, V. (2016) "CMS Grants Navigators $63M to Boost Health Insurance Marketplace." HealthPayerIntelligence. September 8. https://healthpayerintelligence.com/news/cms-grants-navigators-63m-to-boost-health-insurance-marketplace.

[253] Hancock, J. (2019) "UVA Doctors Decry Aggressive Billing Practices by Their Own Hospital." *Kaiser Health News.* November 23, p.1.

[254] Ibid., pp.5–6.

[255] Ibid., p.3.

[256] De Leede, J., and H. Van Laarhoven. (2006) "Lean + at Orbis—How Patient Centered Care and Attractive Workplaces Require Standardised Health Care Processes: Case description, Orbis, for the SALTSA European Hospital Network." Orbis. June, p.8.

[257] Swenson, T. (2020) "The Dark Secret Behind New Hospital Designs." *Op-Med.* February 3.

[258] Smith, D. (2016) "Turnout in the 2016 Elections." *FairVote.* November 16.

[259] Putnam, R. (2000) *Bowling Alone: The Collapse and Revival of American Community.* New York: Simon & Schuster, pp.42–43.

[260] Putnam, R. (2015) *Our Kids: The American Dream in Crisis.* New York: Simon & Schuster.

[261] Ibid., p.240.

[262] Karasek, R. (1979) "Job Demands, Job Decision Latitude, and Mental Strain: Implications for Job Design." *Administrative Science Quarterly* 24 (June), pp.285–308.

[263] Ibid.

[264] Elden, M. (1981) "Political Efficacy at Work: The Connection Between More Autonomous Forms of Workplace Organization and More Participatory Politics." *American Political Science Review* 75, no.1 (March), p.54.

[265] Ibid., p.52.

[266] As the director of the Healthcare Transformation Project at Cornell, I worked closely with Pam Brier and Bruce Richard.

[267] Conversation with Marie-Cecile Charlier, November 30, 2015.

[268] Conversation with Bruce Richard, December 3, 2015.

[269] The Horizons program at Miss Hall's School, in Pittsfield, Massachusetts, requires that their students work three to four hours each week as a volunteer in a community organization to provide them this important civic experience.

[270] Thorsrud, E. (1977) "Democracy at Work: Norwegian Experiences with Non-bureaucratic Forms of Organization." *Journal of Applied Behavioral Science* 13, no.3, p.421.

[271] Cornell consultants were assigned to work with Cook County Health from 2013 to 2014.

[272] Interview with Kris Rondeau, director of the AFSCME New England Organizing Project, June 12, 2018.

[273] Ibid.

[274] Hanleybrown, F., J. Kania, and M. Kramer. (2012) "Channeling Change: Making Collaborative Impact Work." *Stanford Social Innovation Review,* Spring, p.8.

[275] Los Angeles Times. (1991) "UAW Ousts Saturn Union Leader Known for Cooperative Approach." February 25, p. B1.

[276] Hanna, D. (2010) "How GM Destroyed Its Saturn Success." *Forbes.* March 8, pp.1–4.

[277] Ibid., p.2.

[278] Ibid., p.4.

[279] In 2018, several unions that were members of the Coalition of Kaiser Permanente Unions, the umbrella organization representing all participating unions at Kaiser, withdrew from the Coalition and formed their own organization. This organization is called the Alliance of Health Care Unions.

[280] Trahair, R. (2015) *Behavior, Technology, and Organizational Development,* p.253.

[281] Ibid.

[282] Goodman, P.S. (1979) *Assessing Organizational Change: The Rushton Quality of Work Experiment.* New York: John Wiley & Sons.

[283] A Los Angeles County Board of Supervisors resolution on December 12, 2017, created the Labor-Management Transformation Council as a permanent committee of the Los Angeles County Department of Health Services. It allocated yearly funds to continue Labor-Management Partnership activities.

[284] Phone conversation with Jamie Dawson, worksite organizers for Oregon Federation of Nurses and Health Professionals, May 18, 2019.

[285] Bornstein, D. (2007) *How to Change the World: Social Entrepreneurs and the Power of New Ideas.* New York: Oxford University Press, p.291.

[286] Moral Injury Project. (2020) "What Is Moral Injury." Syracuse University, p.1. http://moralinjuryproject.syr.edu.

[287] Shay, Jonathan. (1994) *Achilles in Vietnam: Combat Trauma and the Undoing of Character.* New York: Atheneum.

[288] Dean, W. (2020) "The Real Epidemic: Not Burnout but 'Moral Injury' of Doctors Unable to Do Right by Patients." *WBUR Commentary.* January 24, p.6.

[289] Ofri. (2019) "The Business of Health Care Depends on Exploiting Doctors and Nurses," p.2.

[290] Ibid.

[291] Carey, M.J. (2019) "Time to Address the Widening Pay Gap Between Hospital Execs and Physicians." *Medical Economics* 96, no.8 (April 19), p.2.

[292] Edmondson, A.C. (2019) *The Fearless Organization.*

[293] Brown, T., and S. Bergman. (2020).

[294] Christensen, C.M., J.H. Grossman, and J. Hwang. (2009) *The Innovator's Prescription,* p.192.

[295] Carey, M.J. (2019) "Time to Address the Widening Pay Gap Between Hospital Execs and Physicians."

[296] Shortell, S.M. (2020) "U.S. Health Care System Reform Is Not Yet at the Tipping Point." *To the Point,* Commonwealth Fund. January 14.

[297] Zuger, A. (2017) "Oh, Doctor: The Profit-Driven Disaster That Is U.S. Health Care." Book review. June 13. https://undark.org/2017/06/13/books-rosenthal-american-sickness/.

[298] From Eleanor Roosevelt's speech at the presentation of In Your Hands: A Guide for Community Action for the Tenth Anniversary of the Universal Declaration of Human Rights, March 27, 1958.

References

Abelson, R., and M.S. Sanger-Katz. (2019) "Medicare for All Would Abolish Private Insurance. 'There's No Precedent in American History.'" *New York Times.* March 23, p. A1.

Abrams, M.K. (2014) "Medical Homes: An Evolving Model of Primary Care." *To the Point,* Commonwealth Fund. February 25.

Anderson, I. (1996) "Ethics and Health Research in Aboriginal Communities." In *Ethical Intersections: Health Research, Methods and Researcher Responsibility,* edited by Jeanne Daly. Sydney, Australia: Allen & Unwin Press, pp.513–65.

Appelbaum, E., and L. Hunter. (2004) "Union Participation in Strategic Decisions of Corporations." In *Emerging Labor Market Institutions for the Twenty-First Century,* by R.B. Freeman, J. Hersch, and L. Michel. Chicago: University of Chicago Press.

Baily, M.N., and R.Z. Lawrence. (2004) "What Happened to the Great U.S. Job Machine? The Role of Trade and Electronic Offshoring." Washington, DC. *Brookings Papers on Economic Activity* 2, pp.211–84.

Bandolm, L. (2018) "Study: Almost Half of New Cancer Patients Lose Their Entire Savings." *Insider.* October 23.

Baum, F., C. MacDougall, and D. Smith. (2006) "Participatory Action Research." *Journal of Epidemiology and Community Health* 60, no.10 (October), pp.854–57.

Bellow, H. (2020) "Protective Gear in Short Supply, Says BMC Nurses." *Berkshire Eagle.* March 24, p.1.

Bion, W.R. (1961) *Experiences in Groups: And Other Papers.* New York: Basic Books.

Bluestone, I. (1976) "A Changing View of Union-Management Relations." *Vital Speeches.* December 11.

Bognar, S., and J. Reichert. (2019) "'American Factory': When a Chinese Company Takes Over an Ohio Factory." Washington, DC: High Ground Productions and Netflix. NPR. org, August 21, 2019.

Bornstein, D. (2007) *How to Change the World: Social Entrepreneurs and the Power of New Ideas.* New York: Oxford University Press.

Brooks, D. (2018) "What the Working Class Is Still Trying to Tell Us and How We Can Make a Difference in Their Lives." *New York Times.* November 8, p. A29.

Brown, T. (2015) *The Shift: One Nurse, Twelve Hours, Four Patients' Lives.* Chapel Hill, NC: Algonquin Books of Chapel Hill.

Brown, T. (2018) "Fixing American's Health Care System." *American Journal of Nursing* 118, no.11 (November), p.62.

Brown, T. (2020) "The Reason Hospitals Won't Let Doctors and Nurses Speak Up." *New York Times.* April 21. https://www.nytimes.com/2020/04/21/opinion/coronavirus-doctors-nurses-hospitals.html?searchResultPosition=1.

Carey, M.J. (2019) "Time to Address the Widening Pay Gap Between Hospital Execs and Physicians." *Medical Economics* 96, no.8 (April 19), p.2.

Churchill, W. (1946) Commencement Address at University of Miami.

Christensen, C.M., J.H. Grossman, and J. Hwang. (2009) *The Innovator's Prescription: A Disruptive Solution for Health Care.* New York: McGraw-Hill.

Collins, J. (2005) *Good to Great and the Social Sectors: Why Business Thinking Is Not the Answer.* New York: HarperCollins.

Colman, A., and M. Geller, eds. (1985) *Group Relations Reader 2.* Washington, DC: A.K. Rice Institute.

Dean, W. (2020) "The Real Epidemic: Not Burnout but 'Moral Injury' of Doctors Unable to Do Right by Patients." *WBUR Commentary.* January 24, pp.1–7.

Dolan, T. (2008) "Newark and Its Gateway Complex, Part 3: A Weakened City." *Newark Metro, Rutgers Online.* http://www.newarkmetro.rutgers.edu/reports/display.php?id=17&page= 3; accessed May 25, 2019.

Edmondson, A.C. (2012) *Teaming: How Organizations Learn, Innovate, and Compete in the Knowledge Economy.* San Francisco: Jossey-Bass.

Edmondson, A.C. (2019) *The Fearless Organization: Creating Psychological Safety in the Workplace for Learning, Innovation, and Growth.* Hoboken, NJ: John Wiley and Sons, Inc.

Einstein, A. (1975) Presentation at the *North American Wildlife and Natural Resources Conference,* Wildlife Management Institute, Volume 71, p.54.

Einstein, A. (2010) *The Ultimate Quotable Einstein,* edited by A. Calaprice. Prince ton, NJ: Prince ton University Press, p.474.

Eisold, K. (2010) *What You Don't Know You Know: Our Hidden Motives in Life, Business, and Everything Else.* New York: Other Press.

Elden, M. (1981) "Political Efficacy at Work: The Connection Between More Autonomous Forms of

Workplace Organization and More Participatory Politics." *American Political Science Review* 75, no.1 (March), pp.42–58.

Elden, M., and M. Levin. (1991) "Cogenerative Learning: Bringing Participation into Action Research." In *Participatory Action Research,* edited by W.F. Whyte. Newbury Park, CA: Sage Publications, pp.127–43.

Emery, F.E., and E. Thorsrud. (1969) *Form and Content in Industrial Democracy.* London, UK: Tavistock Institute.

Emery, F.E., and E. Thorsrud. (1976) *Democracy at Work: The Report of the Norwegian Industrial Democracy Program.* Leiden, the Netherlands: H.E. Stenfert Kroese.

Fisher, R.L. (2020) "A Primary Care Physician at His Peak Is Forced into Early Retirement." *MedPage Today.* January 6, pp.1–2.

Freeman, R., and J. Rogers. (1999) *What Workers Want.* Ithaca, NY: Cornell University Press.

Gaille, B. (2017) "21 Incredible Simon Mainwaring Quotes." @Brandongaille.com. May 10, quote number 5.

Gesulga, J., A. Berjame, K.S. Moquiala, and A. Galido. (2017) "Barriers to Electronic Health Record System

Implementation and Information System Resources: A Structured Review." *Procedia Computer Science* 124 (2017), pp.544–51.

Givan, R.K. (2016) *The Challenge to Change: Reforming Health Care on the Front Line in the United States and United Kingdom.* Ithaca, NY: ILR Press/Cornell Press.

Goodman, P.S. (1979) *Assessing Organizational Change: The Rushton Quality of Work Experiment.* New York: John Wiley & Sons.

Greenberg, P.D., and E.M. Glaser. (1980) "Some Issues in Joint Union-Management Quality of Worklife Improvement Efforts." *PsycCRI-TIQUES* 25, no.12 (May), pp.1–95.

Green house, S. (2019) *Beaten Down, Worked Up: The Past, Pre sent, and Future of American Labor.* New York: Alfred A. Knopf, pp.96–97.

Guest, R.H. (1979) "Quality of Work Life—Learning from Tarrytown." *Harvard Business Review,* sec. 57 (July), pp.15–28.

Gustafson, J., and L. Cooper. (1985) "Collaboration in Small Groups: Theory and Technique for the Study of Small Group Processes." In Colman, A., and M. Geller, eds. *Group Relations Reader 2,* pp.139–50. Washington, DC: A.K. Rice Institute.

Gustavsen, B. (2003) "New Forms of Knowledge Production and the Role of Action Research." *Action Research* 1, no.2, pp.153–64.

Hackman, J.R., and G.R. Oldham. (1980) *Work Redesign.* Reading, MA: Addison-Wesley.

Hanleybrown, F., J. Kania, and M. Kramer. (2012) "Channeling Change: Making Collaborative Impact Work." *Stanford Social Innovation Review,* January 26, p.8.

Hanna, D. (2010) "How GM Destroyed Its Saturn Success." *Forbes.* March 8, pp.1–4.

Hayward, S.G., B.C. Dale, and V.C.M. Frazer. (1985) "Quality Circle Failure and How to Avoid It." *European Management Journal* 3, no.2, pp.103–11.

Hersey, P., and K. Blanchard. (1996) *Management of Organizational Behavior: Utilizing Human Resources.* Englewood Cliffs, NJ: Prentice Hall.

Herzberg, F. (1968) "One More Time: How Do You Motivate Employees?" *Harvard Business Review,* pp.46–57.

Hevesi, D. (2007) "Irving Bluestone, 90, Top U.A.W. Negotiator, Dies." *New York Times.* November 21.

Hopper, E. (2003) "The Fourth Basic Assumption: Incohesion: Aggregation/Massification or (ba) I:A/M."

In *Traumatic Experience in the Unconscious Life of Groups,* edited by E. Hopper. London, UK: Jessica Kingsley Publishers, pp.91–107.

Hulin, C.L., and M.R. Blood. (1968) "Job Enlargement, Individual Differences, and Worker Responses." *Psychological Bulletin* 69, no.1, pp.41–55.

Huzzard, T., D. Gregory, and R. Scott, eds. (2004) *Strategic Unionism and Partnership—Boxing or Dancing?* New York: Palgrave Macmillan.

Institute of Medicine and Committee on Quality in Health Care in America. (2001) *Crossing the Quality of Chasm: A Health System for the 21st Century.* Washington, DC: National Academy Press.

Janus v. AFSCME Supreme Court decision (2018). June 27.

Kaës, R. (2007) *Linking, Alliances, and Shared Space: Groups and the Psychoanalyst.* New York: International Psychoanalytical Association

Kania, J., and M. Kramer. (2011) "Collective Impact." *Stanford Social Innovation Review,* Winter, pp.20–29.

Kania, J., and M. Kramer. (2013) "Embracing Emergence: How Collective Impact Addresses Complexity." *Stanford Social Innovation Review.* January 21, pp.1–7.

Kaplan, S. (2012) *Leapfrogging: Harness the Power of Surprise for Business Breakthroughs.* San Francisco: Berrett-Koehler Publishers.

Karasek, R. (1979) "Job Demands, Job Decision Latitude, and Mental Strain: Implications for Job Design." *Administrative Science Quarterly* 24 (June), pp.285–308.

Kernberg, O. (1998) *Ideology, Conflict, and Leadership in Groups and Organizations.* New Haven, CT: Yale University Press.

Klingel, S., and A. Martin. (1988) *A Fighting Chance: New Strategies to Save Jobs and Reduce Costs.* Ithaca, NY: ILR Press/Cornell University Press.

Kochan, T.A., A.E. Eaton, R.B. McKersie, and P.S. Adler. (2009) *Healing Together: The Labor-Management Partnership at Kaiser Permanente.* Ithaca, NY: ILR Press/Cornell University Press.

Kristof, N. (2020) "'I Do Fear for My Staff,' A Doctor Said. He Lost His Job." *New York Times.* April 1. https://www.nytimes.com/2020/04/01/opinion/coronavirus-doctors-protective-equipment.html.

Lazes, P., and A. Costanza. (1984) "Xerox Cuts Costs Without Layoffs Through Union-Management Collaboration." U.S. Department of Labor—Bureau of Labor-Management Relations and Cooperative Program.

Cornell University ILR School. *Policy & Issue Briefs* (July), pp.1–7.

Lazes, P. (1985) "Innovative Approaches to Saving and Creating Jobs." *National Productivity Review* (Spring), pp.146–54.

Lazes, P. (1986) "Employee Involvement Activities: Saving Jobs and Money Too." *New Management* 3, no.3 (Winter), pp.58–60.

Lazes, P., L. Katz, and M. Figueroa. (2012) *How Labor-Management Partnerships Improve Patient Care, Cost Control, and Labor Relations.* Washington, DC: American Rights at Work.

Lazes, P., S. Gordon, and S. Samy. (2012) "Excluded Actors in Patient Safety." In *First Do Less Harm: Confronting the Inconvenient Problems of Patient Safety,* edited by R. Koppel and S. Gordon. Ithaca, NY: ILR Press/Cornell University Press, pp.93–122.

Lazes, P., N. Gregg, and D. Gamble. (2013) *Worker Voice, Unions and Economic Development.* New York: Ford Foundation.

Lazes, P., L.H. Kaplan, and K.A. Gordon. (1987) *The Handbook of Health Education,* 2nd ed. Rockville, MD: Aspen Publishers.

Lazes, P., and J. Savage. (2000) "Embracing the Future: Union Strategies for the 21st Century." *Journal for Quality and Participation* 23, no.4 (Fall), pp.18–23.

Lewin, K. (1951). *Resolving Social Conflicts and Field Theory in Social Science.* New York: Harper and Brothers.

Lewin, K., and D. Cartwright Lewin. (1951) *Field Theory in Social Science: Selected Theoretical Papers.* New York: Harper & Brothers.

Los Angeles County Health Agency Just Culture Policy. (2017) August 14.

Los Angeles Times. (1999) "UAW Ousts Saturn Union Leader Known for Cooperative Approach." February 25, p. B1.

Maimonides Medical Center. (2007) "Creating Competitive Advantage in a Changing Health Care Environment through Worker Participation: Strategic Alliance Report 2007." Brooklyn, NY: Maimonides Medical Center.

Maslow, A. (1954) *Motivation and Personality.* New York: Harper & Row.

McClelland, D.C. (1985) *Human Motivation.* Glenview, IL: Scott, Foresman.

McLeod, A.D., P. Lillrank, and N. Kano. (1991) "Continuous Improvement: Quality Control Circles in Japanese Industry." *Journal of Asian Studies* 50, no.2, p.416.

Nembhard, I.M., J.A. Alexander, T.J. Hoff, and R. Ramanujam. (2009) "Why Does the Quality of Health Care Continue to Lag? Insights from Management Research." *Academy of Management Perspectives* (February), pp.24–42.

Newsweek. (2009) "How GM Crushed Saturn." April 3.

Ofri, D. (2019) "The Business of Health Care Depends on Exploiting Doctors and Nurses." *New York Times.* June 8.

Ovretveit, J., P. Bate, P. Cleary et al. (2002) "Quality Collaboratives: Lessons from Research." *Quality and Safety in Health Care* 11, no.4, pp.345–51.

Parnass, L. (2018) "BMC Nurses Call New Strike, Prompting Hospital to Pull 'Generous' Offer." *Berkshire Eagle,* Pittsfield, MA. June 5, p.24.

Perez, T. (2014) "Using the Workforce as an Engine for Innovation." *Pittsburgh Post Gazette.* June 12, p.24.

Putnam, R. (2000) *Bowling Alone: The Collapse and Revival of American Community.* New York: Simon & Schuster.

Putnam, R. (2015) *Our Kids: The American Dream in Crisis.* New York: Simon & Schuster.

Putnam, R.D., and L.M. Feldstein. (2003) *Better Together: Restoring the American Community.* New York: Simon & Schuster.

Rae-Dupree, J. (2009) "Disruptive Innovation, Applied to Health Care." *New York Times.* February 1.

Reid, R., K. Coleman, E. Johnson, P. Fishman et al. (2010) "The Group Health Medical Home at Year Two: Cost Savings, Higher Patient Satisfaction, and Less Burnout for Providers." *Health Affairs* 29, no.5 (May), pp.835–43.

Reid, T.R. 2009. *The Healing of America: A Global Quest for Better, Cheaper, and Fairer Health Care.* New York: Penguin Press.

Reuther, W. (1941) *500 Planes a Day.* Pamphlet. American Council on Public Affairs, 1941.

Richard, B. (2015) *The Other New York: A Story About Human Transformation.* Kingston, NY: Bruce Richard.

Rolf, D. (2018) *A Roadmap to Rebuilding Worker Power.* New York: The Century Foundation.

Roosevelt, E. (1958) *In Your Hands: A Guide for Community Action for the Tenth Anniversary of the Universal Declaration of Human Rights.* March 27.

Rubinstein, S., and T. Kochan. (2001) *Learning from Saturn: Possibilities for Corporate Governance and Employee Relations.* Ithaca, NY: ILR Press/Cornell University Press.

Rudden, M., S. Twemlow, and S. Ackerman. (2008) "Leadership and Regressive Group Processes: A Pi lot Study." *International Journal of Psychoanalysis* 89, no.5 (November), pp.993–1010.

Rudden, M., P. Lazes, and J. Neumann. (2013) "The Impact of Social Hierarchies on Efforts at Organizational Change: Comparing Two Approaches from the Tavistock Institute for Human Relations." *International Journal of Applied Psychoanalytic Studies* 10, no.3, pp.267–84.

Sandberg, A. (1994) "Volvoism at the End of the Road? Does the Closing-Down of Volvo's Uddevalla Plant Mean the End of Human-Centered Alternative to a Toyotism?" *The Swedish Center for Working Life.*

Sanger-Katz, M. (2019) "Health Costs Are Way Out of Line with the World's." *New York Times.* December 28, p. B1.

Scheiber, N. (2019) "Workers Chase Spoils of Boom on Picket Lines." *New York Times.* October 20, p.20.

Schein, E.H., and P.A. Schein. (2018) *Humble Leadership: The Power of Relationships, Openness, and Trust.* San Francisco: Berrett-Koehler Publishers.

Schiller, B. (1977) "Industrial Democracy in Scandinavia." *Annals of the American Academy of Political and Social Science,* no.431 (May), pp.63–73.

Schwartz, R. (2006) *The Legal Rights of Union Stewards,* 4th ed. Chicago: Labor Notes.

Shapiro, R. (1991) "Psychoanalytic Theory of Groups and Organizations." *Journal of the American Psychoanalytic Association* 39, pp.759–82.

Shay, J. (1994) *Achilles in Vietnam: Combat Trauma and the Undoing of Character.* New York: Atheneum.

Sieden, L.S. (2000) *Buckminster Fuller's Universe: His Life and Work.* New York: Perseus Book Group.

Smith, A. (2014) "The Lucas Plan: What Can It Tell Us About Democratizing Technology Today?" *The Guardian.* January 22.

Smith, D. (2016) "Turnout in the 2016 Elections." *FairVote,* November 16.

Swenson, T. (2020) "The Dark Secret Behind New Hospital Designs." *Op-Med.* February 3.

Taylor, L.K. (1973) "Worker Participation in Sweden." *Industrial and Commercial Training* 5, no.1 (January), pp.6–15.

Thorsrud, E. (1977) "Democracy at Work: Norwegian Experiences with Non-bureaucratic Forms of Organization." *Journal of Applied Behavioral Science* 13, no.3, p.421.

Trahair, R. (2015) *Behavior, Technology, and Organizational Development: Eric Trist and the Tavistock Institute.* New Brunswick, NJ: Transaction Publishers.

Trist, E. (1981) *The Evolution of Socio-technical Systems: A Conceptual Framework and an Action Research Program.* Toronto, Canada: Ontario Quality of Working Life Centre.

Trist, E., and H. Hurray. (1990) *The Social Engagement of Social Science: A Tavistock Anthology.* London, UK: Free Association Books.

Tucker, A.L., A.C. Edmondson, and S. Spear. (2001) "Front-Line Problem Solving: The Responses of Hospital Nurses to Work System Failures." *Academy of Management Proceedings* 2001, no.1, pp. C1– C6.

Tucker, A. L, S.J. Singer, J.E. Hayes, and A. Falwell. (2008) "Front-Line Staff Perspectives on Opportunities for Improving the Safety and Efficiency of Hospital Work." *Health Services Research* 43, no.5, part 2 (October), p.1826.

Twemlow, S., and F. Sacco. (2013) "How and Why Does Bystanding Have Such a Startling Impact on the Architecture of School Bullying and Violence?" *International Journal of Applied Psychoanalytic Studies* 10, no.3, pp.289–306.

U.S. Bureau of Labor Statistics. (2018) *Union Members 2017—Union Member Summary.* January 19.

U.S. Census Bureau. (2018) *Income, Poverty and Health Insurance in the United States: 2017.*

U.S. Senate Subcommittee on Employment, Manpower and Poverty. July 25, 1972.

Walton, R.E. (1973) "Quality of Working Life: What Is It?" *Sloan Management Review* 15, no.1, pp.11–21.

Walston, S.L., P. Lazes, and P.G. Sullivan. (2004) "Improving Hospital Restructuring: Lessons Learned." *Health Care Management Review* 29, no.4, pp.1–12.

Weisbord, M. (2004) *Productive Workplaces Revisited: Dignity, Meaning, and Community in the 21st Century.* San Francisco: Jossey-Bass.

Weisbord, M., and S. Janoff. (2000) *Future Search: An Action Guide to Finding Common Ground in Organizations and Communities.* San Francisco: Berrett-Koehler Publishers.

Whyte, W.F., ed. (1991) *Participatory Action Research.* Newbury Park, CA: Sage Publications, Inc.

Winby, S. (2017) *Sociotechnical Digital Design.* USC Marshall Center for Effective Organizations, April, pp.1–30.

Winby, S., and C.G. Worley. (2014) "Management Processes for Agility, Speed, and Innovation." *Organizational Dynamics* 43, no.3, pp.225–34.

Worley, C.G., S.A. Mohrman, and J.A. Nevitt. (2011) "Large Group Interventions: An Empirical Field Study of Their Composition, Process, and Outcomes." *Journal of Applied Behavioral Science* 47, no.4, pp.404–31.

Acknowledgments

Over the years, several important advisors, mentors, and friends have encouraged Dr. Lazes to pursue his passion for helping union and management leaders involve frontline staff in strategic decision making. Some of those who have helped me on this journey have been union and management leaders—Pam Brier, Mike Bennett, Neal Bisno, the late Irving Bluestone, Gary Bryner, Patricia Castillo, Marie-Cecile Charlier, Kevin Collins, the late Don Ephlin, the late Doug Fraser, Des Geraghty, Mary Kay Henry, Tony Kallevig, Dr. Mitch Katz, Dr. Toni Lewis, the late Gene McCabe, Wilson Mendez, Matt Merrigan, Nicole Moore, Frank Proscia, the late John Reid, Bruce Richard, David Rolf, Kris Rondeau, Josh Rutkoff, Steve Safyer, Eric Scherzer, the late Jack Sheinkman, Bob Schoonover, Andy Stern, Kelly Trautner, Gilda Valdez, Randi Weingarten, and Zack Zobrist. Each, in his or her own way, has helped me understand how unions can play an important role in protecting the rights of workers while also contributing to change processes that benefit patients and their communities.

Researchers at the Norwegian Work Research Institute, Ragnar Johansen and the late Einar Thorsrud, helped me understand the history of industrial democracy in Europe and the role that employee participation activities play in sustaining an active democracy. Paul Clark, Adrienne Eaton, Amy Edmondson, the late Max

Elden, the late Abraham Maslow, Bill Sonnenstuhl, and Marv Weisbord, important colleagues as well as gifted scholars and practitioners, have been exceedingly generous mentors who have encouraged me during different stages of my career. Their influence on my life, my values, and my thinking cannot be overstated.

At the Cornell School of Industrial and Labor Relations, Maria Figueroa, Jeff Grabelsky, Chris Miller, Jane Savage, and the late William F. Whyte have immeasurably supported my research and educational activities. The late Lois Gray, also at Cornell, was an extremely important colleague and mentor who first encouraged me to join the faculty there. With her help I was able to use the university as a home for exploring the importance of Labor-Management Partnerships and contributing to their development in multiple settings.

Consultants Sid Rubinstein, now deceased, and Stu Winby helped me along the way to more deeply understand the practice and methods involved in au then tic worker participation. Lastly, I want to acknowledge Liana Katz for her help in researching and editing this book. She was an invaluable research assistant throughout the process of its creation.

I also want to thank the workers I have come to know over the years who have inspired me with their deep knowledge and passion for their work.

I, Dr. Rudden, wish to remember the late Professor Sidney Mintz, who ignited my enthusiasm for the study of culture in the Yale Anthropology Department, and the late Dr. Roger Shapiro, who led a Tavistock study group during my psychiatric residency that inspired my later work on leadership and the group experience. Drs. Edward Shapiro, Kenneth Eisold, and Vamik Volkan have been important influences in my ongoing study of group behavior and my understanding of the ways in which organizations are influenced by the larger contexts in which they operate. Dr. Stuart Twemlow helped me to appreciate the role of natural leaders in supporting their organizations and communities.

Pam Brier, the former CEO of Maimonides Medical Center, deserves a huge shout-out for supporting and facilitating my research into leadership and group regressions, as does the International Psychoanalytic Association's Research Program and Grants Committee. I am very grateful to John Clarkin, PhD, who mentored my research, and to Cornell University's School of Industrial and Labor Relations for their sponsorship of it. I also owe a good deal to the late Dr. Manuel Furer and to Dr. Robert Michels for their trenchant insights and their significant contributions to my life, both personal and professional.

I would also very much like to thank my patients, who have taught me more than I ever hoped to know.

Both of us offer special thanks to Drs. Paul Clark, John Markowitz, Barbara Milrod, and Bill Sonnenstuhl, and to Robert Sadin and Eric Scherzer, for their close readings of our manuscript and for their invaluable editorial advice. Finally, we thank Rick Finkelstein, whose artistry in designing our book cover has wowed everyone who has seen it.

About the Authors

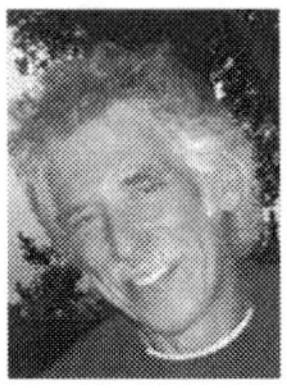

Peter Lazes, PhD, a clinical and industrial psychologist, was the founder and former director of Programs for Employment and Workplace Systems and of the Healthcare Transformation Project, both at Cornell University. He has been an educator, researcher, and practitioner for more than 40 years, dedicated to designing systems in which the knowledge and experience of frontline staff are used to improve patient care and save jobs of American workers. He has written more than 50 articles on engaging frontline staff to improve the effectiveness of their organizations, on leadership, on innovative strategies for improving patient care, and on the importance of meaningful work. He lives with his wife and co-author, Dr. Marie Rudden, in West Stockbridge, Massachusetts.

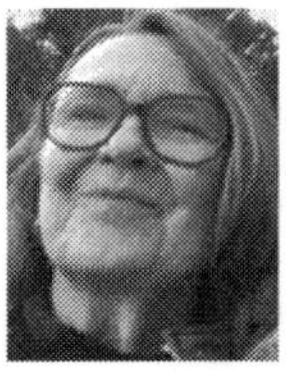

Marie Rudden, MD, a psychiatrist and psychoanalyst, is an associate editor for the *International Journal of*

Applied Psychoanalytic Studies and on the North American Editorial Board of the *International Journal of Psychoanalysis.* A clinical assistant professor in psychiatry at Weill Cornell School of Medicine, she has published widely on panic disorder, depression, leadership in the face of group impasses, and on change processes in psychotherapy. She and her husband, Dr. Peter Lazes, live together with their three horses, mini-donkey, and two dogs in West Stockbridge, Massachusetts.

Berrett–Koehler
BK Publishers

Berrett-Koehler is an independent publisher dedicated to an ambitious mission: *Connecting people and ideas to create a world that works for all.*

Our publications span many formats, including print, digital, audio, and video. We also offer online resources, training, and gatherings. And we will continue expanding our products and services to advance our mission.

We believe that the solutions to the world's problems will come from all of us, working at all levels: in our society, in our organizations, and in our own lives. Our publications and resources offer pathways to creating a more just, equitable, and sustainable society. They help people make their organizations more humane, democratic, diverse, and effective (and we don't think there's any contradiction there). And they guide people in creating positive change in their own lives and aligning their personal practices with their aspirations for a better world.

And we strive to practice what we preach through what we call "The BK Way." At the core of this approach is *stewardship,* a deep sense of responsibility to administer the company for the benefit of all of our stakeholder groups, including authors, customers, employees, investors, service providers, sales partners, and the communities and environment around us.

Everything we do is built around stewardship and our other core values of *quality, partnership, inclusion,* and *sustainability.*

This is why Berrett-Koehler is the first book publishing company to be both a B Corporation (a rigorous certification) and a benefit corporation (a for-profit legal status), which together require us to adhere to the highest standards for corporate, social, and environmental performance. And it is why we have instituted many pioneering practices (which you can learn about at www.bkconnection.com), including the Berrett-Koehler Constitution, the Bill of Rights and Responsibilities for BK Authors, and our unique Author Days.

We are grateful to our readers, authors, and other friends who are supporting our mission. We ask you to share with us examples of how BK publications and resources are making a difference in your lives, organizations, and communities at www.bkconnection.com/impact.

Dear reader,

Thank you for picking up this book and welcome to the worldwide BK community! You're joining a special group of people who have come together to create positive change in their lives, organizations, and communities.

What's BK all about?

Our mission is to connect people and ideas to create a world that works for all.

Why? Our communities, organizations, and lives get bogged down by old paradigms of self-interest, exclusion, hierarchy, and privilege. But we believe that can change. That's why we seek the leading experts on these challenges—and share their actionable ideas with you.

A welcome gift

To help you get started, we'd like to offer you a **free copy** of one of our bestselling ebooks:

www.bkconnection.com/welcome

When you claim your **free ebook,** you'll also be subscribed to our blog.

Our freshest insights

Access the best new tools and ideas for leaders at all levels on our blog at ideas.bkconnection.com.

Sincerely,
Your friends at Berrett-Koehler

Certified B Corporation

A

B

C

D

E

M

X

Printed by Amazon Italia Logistica S.r.l.
Torrazza Piemonte (TO), Italy

10638370R00181